THE
TYPE 2 DIABETES
BREAKTHROUGH

A Revolutionary Approach to Treating Type 2 Diabetes

FRANK SHALLENBERGER, M.D.

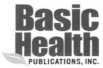

Basic Health
PUBLICATIONS, INC.

The information contained in this book is based upon the research and personal and professional experiences of the author. It is not intended as a substitute for consulting with your physician or other healthcare provider. Any attempt to diagnose and treat an illness should be done under the direction of a healthcare professional.

The publisher does not advocate the use of any particular healthcare protocol but believes the information in this book should be available to the public. The publisher and author are not responsible for any adverse effects or consequences resulting from the use of the suggestions, preparations, or procedures discussed in this book. Should the reader have any questions concerning the appropriateness of any procedures or preparation mentioned, the author and the publisher strongly suggest consulting a professional healthcare advisor.

Basic Health Publications, Inc.
28812 Top of the World Drive
Laguna Beach, CA 92651
949-715-7327

Library of Congress Cataloging-in-Publication Data

Shallenberger, Frank.
    Diabetes breakthrough : a revolutionary approach to treating Type 2
diabetes / Frank Shallenberger.
        p. cm.
    Includes bibliographical references and index.
    ISBN-13: 978-1-59120-126-7 (alk. paper)
    ISBN-10: 1-59120-126-8
    1. Diabetes—Popular works. 2. Insulin—Popular works. I. Title.

    RC660.4.S435   2006
    616.4'62—dc22

                                    2005028053

Copyeditor: Tara Durkin
Typesetting/Book design: Gary A. Rosenberg
Cover design: Mike Stromberg

Printed in the United States of America

10   9   8   7   6   5

Contents

Acknowledgments

Writing a book like this one, with original content and ideas, has been an extremely time-consuming process. More time is spent just in thinking and theorizing than in actual writing, and without the backup and help of many people, this book and the concepts in it may never have had the time to happen.

To my beautiful wife who for so long has put up with the blank looks of a husband whose mind was all too often somewhere else, or who couldn't find the papers that he has been leaving all over the house because some nameless person put them away God only knows where, I apologize and promise to be better. Thank you for your patience, your kindness, and your support for my work. You have made me want to be a better man.

To my staff, the ever trustworthy Robin, the incredibly efficient Melissa, the always-there Tracey, the even-tempered Marcy, the unbelievable Jolene, the dependable Patty, and my ever-so-tidy nurse practitioner and right arm Sheila, this book would have been impossible if you guys were not the greatest.

A very special acknowledgment also needs to go out to my editors at Basic Health Publishing, including copyeditor Tara Durkin, whose remarkable talents were responsible for converting an unintelligible manuscript into something I actually enjoyed reading.

To Tiffany Van der Stoker, who after first inspiring me to write this book then proceeded to write the foreword. My long conversations with you really helped to solidify many of the ideas in this book.

And finally to the Sierra Nevadas and the Nameless Force that moves all things and events and without which nothing good is possible, I love you.

Foreword

WOW! I have been on Dr. Shallenberger's comprehensive type 2 diabetes program for almost two years, and the changes have been nothing short of miraculous!

I am not only bursting with energy, but glowing with vitality and health, not to mention increased stamina *and* no more sleepless nights. Something else I have been able to accomplish as a result of this program is a complete normalization of my blood sugar levels.

As the Executive Secretary of the Nevada State Homeopathic and Integrative Medical Association, I have known Dr. Shallenberger for a good many years. He is and has always been a warrior for the health and well-being of his patients, utilizing natural methods, clean foods, and one's own body's ability to heal itself. He studies continuously and works hard to always be ready to help those who are fortunate enough to find their way to his door.

It seems that traditional Western medicine is and has been for years dependant on artificial means, that is, drugs, which usually mask the problem, have side effects, and do not really heal you. More and more people are falling prey to cancer, type 2 diabetes, strokes, asthma, and many other debilitating illnesses. The numbers grow year by year. The old approach of treating the symptoms while ignoring the cause has never been more popular than it is today. This is not to say that there is no place in our society for pharmaceuticals, but the mass overdosing that goes on is uncalled for, and extremely damaging to our bodies.

Dr. Shallenberger, on the other hand, works with your own body to prevent and/or heal the illness. Type 2 diabetes is absolutely preventable and certainly is curable in many cases. (I believe it is totally curable in all cases given a proper attitude and medical help.) Dr. Shallenberger's methods utilize an innovative test that he has personally developed called Bio-Energy Testing, and an easy protocol, which I am happy to say is responsible for my astonishing success story.

Ultimately, I believe that each one of us is responsible for our own life and our own health. But it's all too typical that for the first thirty to fifty years of our lives we often take so much for granted. Then, when things begin to go wrong and we start to lose that high energy and invulnerable feeling we once had, and when one memorable day we find out that unbeknownst to us we were busy developing diabetes all those years, then things start to change. We start to wonder what we were doing wrong, and whether we can get back on track and regain the health we lost.

Unfortunately, finding the right information and the right doctor to help is not nearly as easy as it ought to be. We usually go to our regular doctor. The same one we have always gone to. The same one who watched over us while we were gaining weight, getting out of shape, and stressing out, and who all too often just said, "Well, Tiffany, looks like we will need to keep an eye on this." What kind of logic is that? Who wants to just keep an eye on the factors that lead to diabetes when changing them can prevent the disease in the first place?

And, then, when we finally are diagnosed, instead of addressing the factors that lead to the disease, all too often we just get a drug to take once or twice a day for the rest of our lives. We are told that diabetes is genetic, and that there is nothing else we can do besides take the medications, follow the American Diabetic Association diet, and wait around to see if we develop the possible consequences of the disease, such as amputation, blindness, kidney failure, or heart disease. Not to mention, we are told that decreased energy and vitality is "inevitable."

I guess I used to be just like the average person who naively thought that all doctors basically did the same thing. That anything and everything that was worth knowing was taught in medical school. And that if it wasn't taught in medical school it was just folklore. I used to be that way, but not anymore!

Whenever I reflect on the fact that each one of us is given just so many days here on this earth, I realize that I want my days and yours, too, to be filled with energy and glowing with health. As Dr. Shallenberger has often told me, "Tiffany, it's just a question of going to the well. I'll lead you there. All you have to do is drink, and the only thing that matters is whether or not you want it enough."

I definitely want it enough, and I am betting, that you do, too! So step into Dr. Shallenberger's parlor, so to speak, and *thoughtfully* read through the pages of this incredible book. The life you save may be your own.

Tiffany Van der Stokker
Reno, Nevada
August 2005

Diabetes Is Preventable and Curable

As I see it every day you do one of two things:
build health or produce disease in yourself.
—ADELLE DAVIS, AUTHOR AND NUTRITIONAL PIONEER (1904–1974)

I t is everyone's greatest desire to have boundless energy and health. Think back to when you were at your healthiest and most energetic; your mind was quick and sharp, positive and unstoppable. What if you could have that back, maybe even better than your best, and keep it for as long as you live? Or maybe you have never felt as vital as you thought you could. Well, this book will educate and guide you to a whole new you.

So what does it take to stay healthy and free of symptoms and disease? If you ask me, it's all about energy— how to keep it if you've got it, and how to get it if you don't. Only by maintaining high energy levels can you stay well, free from disease, young, vibrant, and alive for all the days of your life.

I have spent the last twenty-five years of my professional life searching for answers to why we lose our energy, why we become ill, and even why we age. This research has led me to develop a special interest in one of the most common diseases of these modern times—diabetes, more specifically, type 2 diabetes. Much of this interest has been born from sheer necessity. Due to the fact that the incidence of diabetes is rising so swiftly, like other physicians, I have been seeing an ever-increasing number of patients with this disease.

Approximately 17 million Americans have already been diagnosed with type 2 diabetes, and 16.4 million more have the disease but have not yet been diagnosed. And what could be worse than this? How about the fact that type 2 diabetes, once also known as adult-onset diabetes because it only occurred in adults, is now showing up at an alarming rate in children!

In an article that appeared in *Reuters Health* in 2000, Dr. Gerald Bernstein, a past president of the American Diabetes Association (ADA) was quoted as saying, "If you go back 20 years, about 2% of all cases of new onset diabetes (type 2) were in people between 9 and 19 years old. Now, it's about 30% to 50%."[1] A study published in the March 2002 edition of the *New England Journal of Medicine* looked at a group of obese children and found that 25 percent of them already had a condition that leads to diabetes. And in a June 24, 2003, *USA Today* article, it is estimated that in some ethic groups the rate of childhood type 2 diabetes is approaching over 50 percent![2]

This means that type 2 diabetes is fast approaching epidemic proportions. There are some estimates that at this rate, by the year 2020, more than half of all Americans will have type 2 diabetes.

These are especially staggering numbers considering that the *New England Journal of Medicine* says that type 2 diabetes is 60 percent preventable. So, besides buying stock in companies that cater to the treatment of diabetes, use the information in this book to make sure that you are in the 40 percent without the disease.

My experiences over the years have led me to believe that the unique approach to both the treatment and prevention of this deadly disease, which is discussed in these pages, offers hope. Hope not only to all those people who are living with diabetes today, but also to those who can use these insights to prevent ever getting the disease in the first place. In the following chapters, I will describe how my twenty-plus years of research and clinical experience with thousands of patients has led me to the conclusion that type 2 diabetes is, in fact, an "energy deficit disease."

"An energy deficit disease?" you say, "I have never heard of such a concept. What could he possibly be talking about?" As you will see, what I am talking about is an entirely new way of looking at what causes diabetes. It is an approach that has been overlooked for years because, until recently, we did not have a way of measuring energy production. It is an approach that acknowledges that a decrease in energy production precedes every single case of type 2 diabetes by years, and that this decrease in energy production is precisely what ultimately leads to the expression of the disease. Furthermore, once you grasp the concept that type 2 diabetes is caused by a decrease in energy production, you will easily be able to understand how a comprehensive approach, which is entirely geared at increasing energy production, is so much more effective than the rather myopic view that conventional medicine still offers.

Although this book specifically addresses type 2 diabetes, it is important to note that the same principles are equally effective for type 1, insulin-dependent diabetes.

If you have type 2 diabetes, your physician may have told you that it is genetic, and that there is nothing you can do about it except resign yourself to a lifetime of medication. Similarly, if you have inherited the genes for type 2 diabetes, you might believe that developing the disease is inevitable. The fact is that proclamations such as these are simply not true.

You see, I completely disagree with the *New England Journal of Medicine*'s statement that type 2 diabetes is 60 percent preventable. I believe that it is 100 percent preventable. Not only that, but I have also found that a great many cases are literally curable if found early enough and treated properly.

Diagnosing type 2 diabetes early on is the first step toward conquering the disease. I hope to convince you that everybody, regardless of whether or not there is a family history of diabetes, should be regularly screened not only for diabetes but also for a condition I refer to as "prediabetes."

By prediabetes, I am referring to specific alterations in a person's energy production that are likely to lead to the development of diabetes, and often occur up to ten years before the disease actually sets in. Simply analyzing your blood sugar is not adequate to diagnose prediabetes, and is often not even enough to diagnose the disease after it is present. In this regard, I will show you why I pay special attention to the most sensitive forms of testing for not only diabetes, but also for prediabetes.

You will see that type 2 diabetes results not from some predetermined genetic inevitability, but rather from a multiplicity of factors that ultimately work together to decrease energy production and fat metabolism. I will then show you how to diagnose and correct each one of these factors and thus stop the disease dead in its tracks.

At the very core of my treatment protocol is a unique perspective on exactly what and how much diabetics should be eating in order to optimize energy production. You will quickly learn why the dietary recommendations espoused by the American Diabetic Association are little more than a recipe for keeping the disease.

Another unique component of this energetic treatment approach is an emphasis on optimizing liver function. The chances are good that your physician has never even discussed the role of liver health with you. Conventional wisdom focuses entirely on the pancreas as the organ responsible for diabetes, but, as I have proven over and over again, the liver is more of an issue in most cases of diabetes than is the pancreas. I do not believe that a patient with diabetes can expect to correct or even control this disease without improving liver function.

Another novel and yet important concept that I have discovered after examining the energy-production characteristics of hundreds of my patients is the significant role that hormones play in both the development and the treatment of diabetes. You will soon discover how the thyroid hormones T3 and T4, the adrenal hormones cortisol and DHEA (dehydroepiandrosterone), a hormone called growth hormone, and the sex hormone testosterone are so critical for optimal control, and why it is so necessary to replace these hormones whenever deficiencies are present.

Of course, modern clinical research has conclusively shown that exercise must be an integral part of any successful prevention or treatment plan for type 2 diabetes, but let me be the first to tell you that not any form of exercise will do. Proper exercise is a very individual thing, and cannot be appropriately prescribed using a cookbook approach. Even though most physicians are aware that the level and extent of exercise can actually be detrimental to their patients if not correctly prescribed, few know how to go about prescribing a personalized exercise program for a diabetic.

My patients are not just told to simply start exercising, they are tested for the exact form and level of exercise that will bring them the results that they are looking for. And it may surprise you to learn that my research has shown that the overwhelming majority of diabetics who exercise are exercising too hard to get well!

And did you know that getting adequate amounts of quality sleep on a regular basis is essential not only for the treatment of diabetes but also in order to prevent it? Read on and I will explain why this is so, and how you do an awful lot to improve your health and blood sugar control simply by lying down and closing your eyes.

Stress is that somewhat illusive concept that we all know is behind virtually every disease out there waiting for us. Why? Quite simply, because stress robs us of energy, and all chronic diseases, even the very process of aging itself, primarily occur as a result of decreased energy production. So, if you want to have optimal energy production, you will just have to look at how stress affects you. In this regard, I will offer you some very powerful insights into what causes stress, and how it can be evaporated—quickly, easily, and painlessly.

Ever hear of oxidative medicine? Probably not, because although this form of medical treatment has been widely practiced throughout both eastern and western Europe, it is still relatively unheard of in the rest of the world. I learned about the technique in the early eighties and I have been successfully using it ever since to battle not only diabetes itself, but also many of the complications of diabetes. How can it be that this natural, safe, and effective technology is such a godsend to so many patients with diabetes? By now you might be guessing the answer. It increases energy production.

And, finally, there is the issue of the two kinds of type 2 diabetes. Most physicians are only aware of one kind of type 2 diabetes, but in fact there are two different versions of the disease, and they should be approached somewhat differently. I will discuss how to determine which kind you are, and how that can change the management approach to your program.

But how is it possible that I can be so sure of all this? How can I diagnose not only if a patient already has type 2 diabetes, but also whether or not he will get it? Why am I so positive that my approach can prevent 100 percent of all cases of type 2 diabetes? The answer is that seven years ago, I developed a patented testing procedure called Bio-Energy Testing. Bio-Energy Testing uses FDA-certified oxygen analysis equipment to measure a patient's energy production. After using this form of analysis on literally hundreds of patients, I was able to come to the conclusion that the ultimate cause of diabetes was a combination of two ingredients: (1) having the genes for it, and (2) decreased energy production. Both factors must be present in order to develop type 2 diabetes.

Therefore, I reasoned that if the central cause of diabetes is decreased energy production, increasing and optimizing energy production would both prevent and reverse the disease. And so I set out to discover how it is that humans make energy, why it is that energy production decreases, and how it can be increased to optimal levels.

Interestingly, much of what I learned in this pursuit has turned out to surprise me, because it seemed to counter what I had learned in medical school. Ultimately, however, it led me to discover some key mistakes that I had been making while strictly using conventional wisdom regarding diabetes.

As soon as I started applying the principles that I learned to increase energy production in my diabetic patients, I quickly discovered a dramatic improvement in my success rate. What you are going to find in this book is the fruit of that research and experience.

I believe very strongly in prevention. After all, who in the world would be satisfied simply to manage a disease that can be prevented in the first place? Those persons who don't know whether they are on the road to diabetes or not (that's all of us!) will learn not only how to get the right testing to diagnose both diabetes and prediabetes, but also even how to determine if a tendency toward diabetes is present. Those who already have diabetes will learn of new techniques to rid themselves of this debilitating disease, and go on to live out their lives filled with energy and youthful vigor.

And here's the really good news. All my learning and experience has taught me that diabetes is not necessarily something you have to live with for the rest of your life. Furthermore, all of the many complications of diabetes are not inevitable. To a great extent, it all comes down to the choices you make. In this book I will explain to you what those choices are, and why they are so critical to how well you survive diabetes. The only question that will remain is, are you willing to do what it takes?

PART I

Understanding Diabetes as an Energy Disorder

CHAPTER 1

The Limitations of the Conventional Approach to Treating Type 2 Diabetes

Where there is an open mind there will always be a frontier.
—CHARLES F. KETTERING, ENGINEER AND INVENTOR (1876–1958)

Usually the first thing out of my patients' mouths when they start working with me is, "Why didn't my other doctor tell me all this?" Suffice it to say that controversy in medicine is just a part of the history of the evolution of medicine. Very few ideas are accepted in medicine without going through at least twenty-five to fifty years of being ignored.

Take the issue of cholesterol and its effects on cardiovascular health, for example. Pretty much everybody accepts today that elevated levels of cholesterol in the blood aren't good, and that it would be better to keep these levels to a minimum. But it wasn't always this way.

The cholesterol theory of heart disease was first proposed more than fifty years ago, yet it has only been since the advent of cholesterol medications in the 1990s that the concept has been taken seriously. Before then, the aggressive approach to cholesterol management that is now accepted as "usual and customary" was only given a modicum of lip service. It took more than half of a century for the average physician to take the idea of lowering cholesterol seriously.

That's just the way it works. Many of the ideas you will be reading about in the pages that follow are not entirely new. They aren't my invention. They just have not been around long enough to pass the test of time for the medical profession. Hopefully this book will spur things along, but until then, much of what you read will just have to remain viewed as "unconventional."

However, I'm sure that most readers would agree that the current conventional approach to diabetes is so myopic and limited in scope that almost any new ideas would be welcome. So let's just begin with a discussion of these limitations.

LIMITATION #1: "IT'S ALL ABOUT THE PANCREAS"

The conventional view of type 2 diabetes centers around the pancreas and the hormone it produces, insulin. The pancreas is an organ in the abdomen that, among other vital functions, secretes various digestive enzymes into the intestines. These enzymes are critical for the proper digestion and assimilation of the foods we eat. Fortunately, this digestive aspect of the pancreas only rarely becomes impaired, and for the most part, works adequately even in elderly persons.

The digestive role of the pancreas is not involved in diabetes. What does become involved, however, are the specialized cells in the pancreas, called the islet cells, which produce the hormone insulin.

After a meal that contains carbohydrate is eaten, the digestive system breaks down the carbohydrate into sugars, and these sugars are then absorbed into the bloodstream and immediately carried to the liver for processing. After the sugars are processed by the liver, they are then released into the bloodstream, causing an elevation of the blood sugar, or glucose, levels.

The elevation in the blood glucose levels is what then stimulates the islet cells of the pancreas to secrete the hormone insulin into the bloodstream. I should mention here that fats and proteins in the diet also result in some insulin secretion, but the amount of insulin secreted is so low that it is inconsequential when compared with the effects of dietary carbohydrate.

Once insulin is secreted into the bloodstream, it interacts with the membranes on all the cells in the body with the one exception of the brain cells. This interaction allows the cells to take up the glucose from the blood. The glucose is then either metabolized into energy or stored as glycogen or fat.

As the body's cells take up the glucose, the blood glucose levels decrease. Conversely, if the pancreas were not able to make enough insulin, the cells of the body would not be able to absorb the elevated levels of glucose that emerge in the blood after a carbohydrate meal, and the blood glucose would go up, resulting in the high blood sugar levels typical of diabetes.

But there are two very different conditions that can cause blood glucose levels to be elevated in type 2 diabetes. And these conditions lead to what I refer to as the two different kinds of type 2 diabetes. The first kind I just mentioned and that happens when the pancreas is not able to make adequate amounts of insulin. In this case, when the blood insulin levels are checked, they are found to be low. I call this the low-insulin kind of type 2 diabetes.

The other condition is the high-insulin kind of type 2 diabetes. High-insulin diabetes involves a condition referred to as insulin resistance. As you will see as you read on, this distinction is quite important when it comes to the treatment of type 2 diabetes. The low-insulin form of diabetes is the worst kind in terms of difficulty treating and amount of complications. It is preceded by the high-insulin form. In fact, it is caused by the high-insulin form. Therefore, by aggressively identifying and treating the high-insulin form, it is possible to prevent the low-insulin form from ever developing.

Insulin resistance happens when the membranes of the cells of the body no longer respond to insulin by taking up glucose. In other words, they become resistant to the effects of insulin. This condition is also referred to as a loss of insulin sensitivity, and I will often use this term interchangeably with insulin resistance. Exactly what causes insulin resistance, or loss of insulin sensitivity, is said to be unknown, but my research into the energy-production mechanisms of the body have led me to believe that it is ultimately a result of an energy deficit (we'll discuss this more in later chapters).

In the case of insulin resistance, the pancreas is making plenty of insulin, but the cells of the body don't respond properly. As a result, the blood glucose levels stay elevated just the same as when there is an insulin deficiency.

Insulin resistance doesn't just happen overnight. It develops slowly over many years, and during this time, since the insulin is not producing the proper response, the islet cells make increasingly greater amounts of insulin in order to keep the blood glucose levels from becoming too high. Thus, a hallmark of insulin resistance is that the blood levels of insulin become quite elevated. Insulin resistance is what causes the high-insulin form of diabetes.

But there is a cost to placing so much demand on the islet cells, and the cost is paid in the form of excessive "free-radical" production. Free radicals are a class of molecules that are an everyday product of energy production in all cells of the body. The more energy that is being produced in a cell, the more free radicals are produced. The production of free-radical molecules is a normal, healthy part of energy metabolism, and islet cells are no exception to this rule.

Remember when I told you that the real problem behind insulin resistance was poor energy production? Well, the excessive production of free radicals is one of the primary reasons. When a cell becomes less and less efficient at producing energy, the amount of free radicals it produces dramatically increases. If the energy-deficient cell is an islet cell being forced to produce ever-increasing amounts of energy in order to manufacture insulin in a patient developing insulin resistance, the production of free radicals increases even more.

Now, the nature of free radicals is such that even though they are a normal part of cellular energy production, when their levels are increased beyond a critical amount, they become highly damaging and will literally destroy the cell that is making them. And eventually, this is the process by which energy inefficient, overworked islet cells come to their certain demise.

This process of free-radical damage, which happens over many years, ultimately destroys so many islet cells that the pancreas, which was once producing excessive amounts of insulin to compensate for insulin resistance, now becomes unable to produce even minimal levels of insulin. When the islet cells can no longer compensate by making more insulin, the blood glucose levels begin to climb and diabetes is diagnosed.

So the conventional concept of type 2 diabetes goes like this: For reasons that are believed to be unknown, many people will develop insulin resistance. As insulin resistance increases and places increasingly greater production demands on the pancreas, the islet cells become slowly destroyed by the action of the free-radical molecules that are produced along with the insulin. Then, as the islet cells become reduced in number, the pancreas is no longer able to make sufficient amounts of insulin, and ultimately an insulin deficiency results. When the insulin deficiency reaches a critically low level, the blood glucose starts to climb and type 2 diabetes is diagnosed.

I believe that these conventional concepts and the treatment strategies that follow from them are way too limited because they do not address several vital issues:

1. What causes insulin resistance in the first place?

2. How can insulin resistance be corrected?

3. How can the pancreas be protected from free-radical damage?

The reason that the conventional perspective of type 2 diabetes is unable to answer these questions is that it only focuses on the pancreas. The function of the entire rest of the body is ignored as if it were not there or played no role whatsoever in the management of blood glucose levels. As you will soon learn in the following pages, this kind of thinking is seriously flawed.

LIMITATION #2: "IT'S ALL ABOUT GENETICS"

The conventional approach to type 2 diabetes places way too much importance on genetics. In fact, many physicians state it very simply, "If you have the genes for type 2 diabetes, you are going to get it, and if you don't you're not." From a scientific perspective, a statement such as this is pure hogwash.

The fact is, if you have the gene for any medical disorder you are statistically more prone to get it, but that doesn't mean that you will. Conversely, there are some forms of type 2 diabetes that are not genetically dependent at all, and are caused simply by poor lifestyle choices. In order to understand how this works, you will need to know the difference between genotype and phenotype.

Your genotype is the genetic code you have, it cannot be changed. Your phenotype is how that genetic code actually gets expressed in your body. The phenotype is determined by lifestyle factors, things that you can change, such as your living conditions, your hygiene, how you eat, play, exercise, sleep, deal with stress, and so on. Even though you may have the genetic code for developing a disease, whether or not you actually get it is determined by whether or not you develop the phenotype for it, and that is established by how you live.

A good example of this distinction is found in patients who are born with a condition called phenylketonuria. Because of a genetic disorder these patients are not genetically able to cope with the amino acid phenylalanine, and they can easily develop serious medical problems if they eat foods high in this amino acid. They have the genotype for these medical conditions, but as long as they eat very little phenylalanine, they will not develop the phenotype, and can go on to leading perfectly healthy lives.

The important message here is that science has shown over and over that an individual's phenotype accounts for about 90 percent of the incidence of any given disease, while the genotype accounts for only about 10 percent. The incidence of type 2 diabetes is an especially good example of this. People with a family history of diabetes need to understand that having the gene for the disease means relatively little. Nine out of ten times, the reason a person gets the disease is not because he or she has the gene for it, but because the person's lifestyle allows the gene to express itself.

I think that this point is critically important because there is a tendency for people with a family background of diabetes to give up or to make excuses for themselves. It's also important because if an individual has a family history of diabetes, he or she should realize that it is even more important to follow the preventive recommendations in this book than it is for someone without that history.

The importance of phenotype over genotype in type 2 diabetes can be readily seen in the simple fact that diabetes was relatively rare a hundred years ago, even though we still have the same basic gene pool that we had then. The recent dramatic increase in the incidence of diabetes is solely a result of the environmental influences on phenotype, and cannot be attributed to genetics. This phenomenon has been well documented in any number of population studies. A good example is the once nomadic tribes of Yemen.

At the turn of the last century, a group of anthropologists examined several nomadic tribes in Yemen and were unable to find any cases of diabetes. However, by the 1930s and 1940s, the tribes had given up their nomadic ways and had settled in metropolitan areas where their lifestyles became markedly different, especially with respect to their eating habits. As a result, they began to show the same incidence of diabetes that is typical of city populations, even though their genetic pool had not changed. This study demonstrates how modern lifestyles have an effect on the phenotypic expression of diabetes.

So just because you have a family history of diabetes doesn't mean you are going to get it. By the same token, however, just because you don't have a family history of diabetes doesn't mean you won't get it. You could easily have had a family member that had the genes for diabetes but either failed to get it because of his or her healthy lifestyle, or because he or she died before it was diagnosed. Tiffany, who was kind enough to write the foreword to this book, is one example. She was recently diagnosed with type 2 diabetes although she has no family history of it ever occurring. She does recall that her grandfather, who was very heavy, had his leg amputated and died of congestive heart failure. It is highly likely that he had diabetes and it was never diagnosed. Consequently, even though it has been there since her birth, Tiffany had no clue that she had the genes for diabetes.

All you really need to know is that diabetes is an energy deficit disorder, and that all that you need to do is to follow the advice in this book and keep your energy levels vibrant and youthful. If you will just do that, no matter what your genes are, you will never have to deal with diabetes.

LIMITATION #3: "IT'S ALL ABOUT TREATMENT"

The third problem with the conventional approach to diabetes is that the focus is on treatment. That modern medicine, pretty much across the board, does little to nothing to prevent disease, is perhaps its greatest deficiency.

This focus on treatment can also be seen in modern medicine's approach to cancer, heart disease, and any other condition you can name, but it is especially noticeable in diabetes. Sadly enough, our society seems to be very satisfied with a medical system that goes blindly along miraculously putting out the fires of disease, while at the same time spending essentially no effort to prevent these fires.

Not only is this approach a travesty to all those persons who needlessly develop preventable diseases, but it is also a sure way to bankrupt our economy. Can you say "higher taxes"? Putting out fires is expensive. Preventing them is cheap.

By prevention, I mean the early detection of prediabetes. By prediabetes, I am referring to a number of metabolic imbalances, often including insulin resistance, which *always* precede diabetes by many years, and which will eventually lead to the development of the disease.

If these imbalances are recognized and treated before the disease develops, all my research indicates that diabetes can be prevented 100 percent of the time. If fully implemented, that would mean that the incidence of type 2 diabetes would be just what it once was among the nomadic tribes mentioned earlier—zero. In Chapter 4, I will show you how prediabetes can be diagnosed, and in the rest of the book I'll be demonstrating how prediabetes can be turned around.

LIMITATION #4: FAILURE TO REALIZE
THAT IT'S REALLY ALL ABOUT ENERGY

In the beginning of this chapter, I mentioned that my research into the energy production mechanisms of the body have led me to believe that insulin resistance and all of the other factors that lead to type 2 diabetes are the result of an energy deficit.

For now let me briefly explain: Every aspect of every function in the human body is dependent on energy production. That means a decrease in energy production in a person with the genetic traits for diabetes can affect a multiplicity of factors that ultimately cause the disease. This is why I refer to type 2 diabetes as an energy deficit disorder.

In my opinion, the single most limiting aspect of the conventional approach to the treatment and prevention of type 2 diabetes is that it doesn't recognize the relationship between decreased energy production and the phenotypic expression of the disease. Because of this limitation, physicians treating diabetes are faced with the following problems:

- They do not appreciate that there are two forms of type 2 diabetes.

- They prescribe the wrong diet.

- They don't understand the value of nutrient supplementation.

- They prescribe incorrect exercise.

- They don't understand the regulating effects of the liver.

- They ignore the effect of sleep debt.

- They don't understand the effects of stress.

- They don't understand the importance of hormones other than insulin.

- They don't understand the therapeutic advantage of oxidative medicine.

- They have no good way to prevent the disease.

Being able to measure the energy production of my patients with Bio-Energy Testing (see Chapter 2) has erased all of the above problems for me. It allows me to be specific regarding my dietary, supplement, and exercise recommendations. It further allows me to provide targeted therapeutics to my patients to optimize the function of their liver. This alone gives me a tremendous advantage.

Additionally, being able to measure and improve energy production has also taught me the importance of regulating stress and ensuring adequate sleep. Most notably, I have learned the value of prescribing hormone replacement therapy when it is indicated.

But perhaps the most significant benefit of treating energy deficits is disease prevention. The decrease in energy production that leads to type 2 diabetes can be diagnosed and treated many years before the disease actually shows up. As long as my patient has optimal energy production, I know he or she will never be bothered with diabetes.

In the next chapter, you'll learn all about this exquisitely sensitive and novel form of testing.

CHAPTER 2

Bio-Energy Testing

The world belongs to the energetic.
—RALPH WALDO EMERSON, ESSAYIST AND POET (1803–1882)

homas Edison, considered by many to be the greatest genius of the twentieth century, once said that the doctor of the future would be much less interested in prescribing medicine to treat a disease than in prescribing measures to prevent it. After more than thirty years of listening to patients describe the ordeals of having a disease that I know is completely preventable, I can't help but wonder just when these doctors of the future are going to show up in significant numbers.

The tragedy of diabetes is certainly a case in point. This is a potentially devastating disease, the cause of which—decreased energy production—can easily be discovered and eliminated long before the disease even begins to take hold. The key is to measure energy production, and that is exactly what Bio-Energy Testing does.

Bio-Energy Testing measures the oxygen and carbon dioxide content of your breath every time you inhale and exhale. It does this using a mouthpiece and FDA-approved measuring devices. Bio-Energy Testing also measures your heart rate, the amount of work you perform on an exercise bicycle, your respiration rate, your percentage of body fat, and your blood pressure. As you will discover in the pages that follow, this simple data can be used to accurately and reliably determine and improve energy production.

Measurements are taken while you are at rest and during an exercise protocol. All of this "breath-by-breath" data is then analyzed by a patented computer program that is able to determine not only your energy production dynamics but also many other important factors about your health.

19

What Bio-Energy Testing Tells You

- How well your body is producing energy
- How well your body metabolizes fat
- Your metabolic rate
- Your adrenal gland function
- Your heart function
- Your lung function
- Your body fat percentage
- Your level of fitness
- Your particular optimal caloric intake
- Your particular optimum carbohydrate intake
- Your optimum exercise parameters
- Your biological age

WHO BENEFITS FROM THE TEST?

Certainly anyone with diabetes is operating from a deficit if they do not have the information provided by the test (see the inset "What Bio-Energy Testing Tells You"). However, although this book is specifically about diabetes, the fact is that Bio-Energy Testing is essential not only for diabetics but also for the following people:

- Anyone interested in slowing down the aging process

- Anyone who wants to feel and function like a much younger person

- Any chronically fatigued individual

- Anyone needing help with weight control

- Anyone interested in preventing the diseases of aging, such as diabetes

- Anyone with heart disease, arthritis, or high cholesterol

- People who want to know if their disease-prevention program is working or not

- Anyone who wants to exercise "smart"

THE TESTING PROCESS

The Bio-Energy Testing process involves a resting phase and an exercise phase. The resting part of the test is performed in the morning usually before 11:30 A.M. You should not eat or drink anything other than water. Be extremely lazy before the test. Both physical and mental exertion should be kept to a minimum, and definitely no exercise.

After you arrive at the testing center, the technician measures and records your body fat percentage, height, and weight. Next, a heart-rate monitor is placed on your chest while you sit in a comfortable reclining chair.

Within a few minutes of settling down in the chair, the technician places a mouthpiece in your mouth. There is no discomfort, so relaxing won't be a problem. As you just lay back and rest, the analyzer determines your oxygen intake, carbon dioxide output, and other vital signs.

After this initial resting measurement, the fun really begins. You are placed on an ergometer, a fancy name for an exercise machine, in this case a bicycle, that uses a computer to measure how hard you are working. The technician again gives you the measuring mouthpiece to place in your mouth. Now you begin to cycle.

For the first several minutes, very little effort is required. Then the workload on the ergometer gradually increases so that you have to work harder to turn the pedals. As the level of exertion increases, your heart rate also increases.

The test continues until the technician notifies you that you have maximized your oxygen consumption, and at this point the test is concluded. The entire process, both the resting and the exercise part, takes about forty-five minutes.

ANALYZING A BIO-ENERGY TESTING REPORT

At this point, let me reintroduce you to Tiffany Van der Stokker. Tiffany is sixty-two years old. She is a wonderful person whom I have known socially and professionally for many years, but who had never been my patient. Among her many talents, Tiffany is a professional writer, and knowing this, I asked her to help me put this book together.

Two years ago, as part of the process of working with me on the book, we decided to put her through the testing process just so she could learn more about it. Well, wouldn't you just know it? Lo and behold, to our surprise and amazement, Tiffany turned out to have type 2 diabetes. For just how many years her case had been undiagnosed we did not know, because up until the last ten to twelve months, she had been feeling as good as she ever had.

In Chapter 14 I will be discussing the details of Tiffany's case, along with what treatment strategies were employed as a result of her Bio-Energy Testing results. But for the purpose of explaining to you how the test actually works, let's go over the results of her very first test. All of the following parameters are determined from Bio-Energy Testing.

Resting Heart Rate

The heart is a muscle, and like any other muscle it can be exercised and strengthened to pump at a maximum level of efficiency. The resting heart rate is a reliable indicator of just how efficiently the heart is pumping. A heart that is pumping efficiently will pump out larger amounts of blood per beat, and thus will need to beat less often in order to pump a given amount of blood. A less-efficient heart would need to beat more often in order to pump out the same amount of blood.

A heart pumping as efficiently as possible will help prevent cardio-vascular disease, and is the key to optimal energy production. The ideal resting heart rate should be below 72 beats per minute. A resting heart rate indicating maximum heart efficiency would be below 65.

Resting heart rates that are greater than 72 may indicate any of the following conditions:

- A poorly conditioned heart

- Excessive thyroid activity

- Failure to fast adequately before the test

- Claustrophobia or test anxiety

Resting heart rates that are lower than 55 may indicate any of the following:

- A highly conditioned heart typical of an athlete

- Thyroid deficiency

- Adrenal insufficiency

- The use of beta-blocker medication

Tiffany's resting heart rate was 70, which is normal.

Resting Respiratory Rate

The resting respiratory rate is a reliable indicator of how efficiently you breathe, as well as how easily you can relax. There are two ways that the body can breathe. One involves using the diaphragm to pull air into the lungs, and is called diaphragmatic or abdominal breathing. This is the most effective way of breathing. The other is by using the chest, shoulder, and neck muscles to elevate the chest wall. This kind of breathing is called chest-wall breathing. Both processes are described in Chapter 11, which discusses stress.

Chest-wall breathing, because it is the most inefficient way to oxygenate the blood, triggers a subtle, but measurable, increase in the breathing rate. This increased breathing rate, due to its effects on the pH of the blood, results in decreased energy production and often causes feelings of anxiety. Chronic chest-wall breathing is also a common cause of neck and shoulder discomfort.

An optimum resting respiratory rate is under seven breaths per minute, but any rate lower than ten is acceptable. Rates above fifteen indicate a significant problem in this area. Tiffany's resting respiratory rate was eleven breaths per minute, which indicated that she could use a little work on her abdominal breathing, but it was not a significant problem for her energy-producing mechanisms.

The Breathing Factor

The Breathing Factor indicates the amount of carbon dioxide that is present in the breath toward the end of each exhalation. Studies have revealed that when a subject has a decreased percentage of carbon dioxide in this portion of the breath, there is a strong likelihood that he or she has chronic hyperventilation syndrome. Chronic hyperventilation syndrome refers to symptoms and conditions that develop as a result of chronic shallow breathing that leads to a subtle increase in the breathing rate.

Besides often causing an exaggerated stress response associated with anxiety, insomnia, and even panic attacks, chronic hyperventilation syndrome also results in decreased energy production. In patients with asthma, chronic hyperventilation can also precipitate asthma attacks.

Normally the optimum range for Breathing Factor is from 100 to 115. A Breathing Factor less than 100 indicates the presence of chronic hyperventilation, and less that 90 indicates a severe condition. Less than 60 is actually life threatening!

Tiffany's Breathing Factor was 105, which indicated that she does not have a problem with chronic hyperventilation syndrome.

The Adrenal Factor

I believe that one of the major factors in decreased energy production is stress. Stress results from external sources such as allergies, infection, pain, chemical exposure, insomnia, and so on, and from internal sources such as anxiety, anger, and so on. All of these various stressors throw our bodies out of balance, and it is the adrenal glands that, by producing the hormones cortisol and DHEA (dehydroepiandrosterone), act to keep us in a state of balance even in the face of continued stress.

Eventually, however, the adrenal glands may become exhausted. When this happens, the body will no longer be able to maintain a healthy state of balance, and energy production will decrease.

The Adrenal Factor is the ratio of the systolic blood pressure while lying down to the same after immediately standing up. An Adrenal Factor greater than 100 indicates a healthy adrenal response. Values less than 100 indicate progressively declining adrenal function.

Treatment for a low adrenal function involves decreasing the sources of stress, combined with taking supplements and hormones to support the adrenal glands. In most cases, with adequate support, the adrenal glands will renew themselves within three to four months of treatment.

Tiffany's Adrenal Factor was 95, which indicated that her adrenal glands were starting to weaken. Low adrenal gland function leads to the single most common complaint doctors hear, "I'm tired. What's wrong with me?"Tiffany had this complaint, and now her Bio-Energy Testing is telling us one of the reasons why.

Her adrenal insufficiency was also verified by examining the levels in her blood of the hormone cortisol, the primary hormone of the adrenal gland, and finding that it was quite low. As you will see in Chapter 12, the hormone cortisol is extremely important in diabetes, because its action is to improve fat metabolism.

The Heart Factor

Just like any other muscle, the heart can lose its muscle mass and become weak as part of the aging process. As it becomes weak, it is unable to pump out as much blood per stroke. As this happens, the heart will have to beat more times per minute in order to deliver the same amount of blood. This means that in order for it to pump out enough blood to meet the body's requirements, the heart will have to beat many more times per minute than a healthy, conditioned heart, resulting in increased oxygen demands and decreased function.

It is this decrease in heart function that is responsible for the incidence of heart failure so commonly seen in the elderly. Furthermore, a decrease in heart function also decreases energy production in *every other organ* in the body because the heart is less able to adequately pump out the body's oxygen requirements.

The scientific literature has established equations that can be used to predict how well anyone's heart should be pumping. By entering the age, weight, sex, and height of an individual into the equations, that person's "predicted" heart-pumping value can be determined. The Heart Factor is the actual measurement of the pumping ability of the heart using Bio-Energy Testing, divided by the "predicted" value. This value is then reported on the test as a percentage of what is predicted for that person.

For example, if the Heart Factor is 135, this means that the subject's heart is pumping about 135 percent of what would be expected for that person. Obviously, that would indicate very good heart function. Likewise, if the Heart Factor were 75, this would indicate that the subject's heart was only pumping about 75 percent of what would be expected. This, of course, represents a poorly functioning heart.

As you continue to read about the other Factors that are reported in Bio-Energy Testing, you will see the same method employed. Each measured value will be compared to the predicted value for that person, and the results will be presented as a percentage of what is predicted. Oh yes, there are two more important distinctions in determining the Factors that you should know about.

When a subject is older than forty, the computer does not enter the subject's actual age into the predicted equation. Instead it always enters the age of forty. Thus for those persons older than forty, the Factors are comparing them to what would be predicted for a person of the same sex, height, and weight who is not their same age, but is forty years old. This is done because forty years old is considered by most anti-aging experts to be when the aging process begins, and I don't want my patients to be "healthy for their age"—I want them to be healthy for any age.

The other change that is made in the prediction equations for all of the Factors that I will be discussing is that the person's weight is corrected for body fat. In other words, if a person is overweight, instead of entering into the equations the person's real weight, the computer enters in the weight that that person would be if he or she were not overweight. This is an important consideration, because it turns out that persons who are overweight are penalized in the equations, and this change corrects for that.

Heart Factor can vary significantly according to genetics, but typically a healthy value is greater than 100. Tiffany's Heart Factor was 86, indicating that her heart was only pumping about 86 percent as well as it was when she was forty. Tiffany's heart was getting weaker. This level of decline did not necessarily mean that her heart was diseased. Rather, in all likelihood it only demonstrated how deconditioned the cardiac muscle had become because she had not been exercising for such a long time. Such a low number was an incentive for Tiffany to start taking better care of her heart.

The Lung Factor

Examining the rate of oxygen intake and carbon dioxide production enables Bio-Energy Testing to accurately determine the lung function. Just as with every other aspect of health, lung function also decreases as a result of aging. Furthermore, it can be compromised by damage to the lungs from cigarette smoke, chemicals, allergies, and infectious diseases.

Since your lungs serve as the exchange site for oxygen to enter your body, adequate lung function is required for optimal energy production. Learning to breathe properly, exercising, and protecting the lungs from smoke and allergies are important ways to improve lung function.

Just like with the Heart Factor, the Lung Factor is a percentage measurement. It is arrived at by dividing how much air a person's lungs can actually hold, known as the "vital capacity," by the predicted vital capacity for that person. And just like with the Heart Factor, if the person is older than forty, the age of forty is entered into the prediction equations, and if the person is overweight a corrected weight is entered.

The Lung Factor value can vary significantly according to genetics. Some people are just born with a much larger vital capacity than others. But typically a healthy value is greater than 100, indicating that the subject's lungs still have youthful function.

Tiffany's Lung Factor was 88. She might have lost a little bit in this department over the years, but I consider this measurement to be basically normal.

Body Composition Analysis

Body composition analysis refers to the percentages of fat and muscle that the body has. It is regarded as an extremely reliable predictor of health and aging. The higher your body fat percentage, the more prone you are to disease across the board. Conversely, the higher your percentage of muscle, the lower your incidence of disease.

Diabetes in particular is adversely affected by a *decrease* in muscle mass and an increase in fat mass. Both of these changes are caused by a decrease in energy production. Here's how it works. Whenever you eat, the food gets converted to fat for storage to be used later for energy production. Therefore, when energy production becomes decreased (because of toxicity, decreased hormone levels, and so on), the stored fat is not used for energy production and over time accumulates. And, because it takes energy to build muscle, low energy production also results in decreased muscle formation. It is these changes that are responsible for the change in physique that commonly occurs with aging, and it is certainly responsible for the significant association between type 2 diabetes and obesity.

An ideal body fat percentage for a woman is between 18 and 22 percent. A person is obese when his or her body fat percentage is greater than 30 percent. Tiffany's body fat percentage was 34 percent, putting her into the obese category and greatly decreasing her body's ability to maintain optimal blood sugar control. She will need to lose about fifty pounds of fat in order to bring her diabetes under control. In order to do that, she will need to have an optimal fat-burning metabolism (we will discuss this in "The C-Factor" below).

The C-Factor

One of the most important pieces of information that comes out of Bio-Energy Testing is the C-Factor. The C-Factor measures how well your body is burning fat in a resting state.

The C-Factor is critical in Tiffany's case, because without an optimal fat-burning metabolism, she will be unable to maintain control over her weight, her energy production will go down, and her cells will be forced to live off glucose. These three conditions are what led her down the road to diabetes in the first place, and failing to correct them will make it impossible for her to adequately treat her condition.

Research has shown that when young, healthy, athletic individuals are at rest they are producing the majority of their energy, at least 75 percent, from fat. This makes complete sense because, as you will learn in the next chapter, the body prefers to burn fat because fat stores are so much more plentiful than carbohydrate stores, and because fat burns cleaner. However, when I measure the C-Factor on a new patient, I usually discover that the patient is producing only about 45 to 50 percent of his or her energy from fat. This finding is very significant because it means that the energy production in these patients is being shifted away from primary fat metabolism to primary glucose metabolism. As you will see, this shift away from fat metabolism plays a major role in the cause of obesity, diabetes, and virtually every other disease, from cancer to fatigue. I believe it is even at the very root of aging itself!

C-Factor measures the percentage of your energy production at rest that comes from fat metabolism. A C-Factor greater than 100 indicates that you are producing at least 75 percent of your resting energy production from fat, which points to optimal resting fat metabolism. A C-Factor less than 100 indicates that you are progressively producing less than 75 percent of your resting energy production from fat, which points to less-than-optimal resting fat metabolism. A C-Factor as low as 50 indicates that you are not producing any resting energy production at all from fat, which points to a severe impairment of fat metabolism. The lower the C-Factor, the greater your potential is for gaining weight.

So why do I call this the C-Factor? Why don't I just call it the Fat-Burning Factor? The reason is very simple. More than any other single factor, resting fat metabolism is suppressed by eating too much carbohydrate. Thus, I call this measurement the C-Factor because it indicates whether or not your diet contains so much carbohydrate that it is interfering with optimal fat burning. A low C-Factor—that is, under 100—indicates that the body's fat metabolism is being hijacked by excessive dietary carbohydrates, particularly middle- and high-glycemic carbohydrates (see "The Glycemic Index" on page 29).

Tiffany's C-Factor was 76, indicating that for her particular physiology, her carbohydrate intake was way over the line. This greatly limits her ability to control her diabetes because it is suppressing her ability to metabolize fat, and in doing so, causes her to rely more on glucose. Tiffany will need to decrease her dietary intake of carbohydrates. How much should the carbohydrate level be cut back? This varies greatly from person to person, but the reduction must be sufficient enough to bring the C-Factor up to 100 or higher. I have found that in the majority of

The Glycemic Index

It is important to stress that some carbohydrates suppress fat metabolism much more than other carbohydrates. The differences are clarified in an indexing system called the glycemic index.

The glycemic index has been determined through experimentation in which subjects are given various carbohydrate-containing foods to eat in order to see how much insulin their bodies produce as a result of eating these foods. The carbohydrate foods that result in the greatest production of insulin are referred to as high-glycemic carbohydrates. Since one of the major actions of insulin is to shut down fat metabolism, the high-glycemic carbohydrates, particularly sugar and flour, are the worst offenders and suppress fat metabolism the most. Those foods that result in the lowest amount of insulin secretion, and hence suppress fat metabolism the least, are classified as low-glycemic carbohydrates. And those foods that fall in the middle are called middle-glycemic carbohydrates.

High-Glycemic Carbohydrates

- Bread (white or whole grain—it makes no difference), pastry, cookies, crackers, pretzels, pancakes, and so on—basically anything that is made from flour with the one exception of pasta.

- Rice (both white and brown), corn, millet, barley, chips, cold breakfast cereals (including muesli), cooked cereals (with the one exception of slow-cooked oatmeal).

- Bananas, pineapple, raisins, melons, mango, papaya, pumpkin.

- All sweets. This means literally anything that tastes sweet, including honey, fruit juices, corn syrup, maple syrup, high-fructose corn syrup, maltose, barley malt, maltodextrin, sugar, and molasses. Always check ingredients labels for sugars. Anything that ends in -ose is a sugar. The exceptions are pure fructose, artificial sweeteners, and the herb stevia.

- All root vegetables, with the one exception of yams. This includes potatoes, carrots, sweet potatoes, beets, and so on.

- Beer and wine (even the low alcohol kind). All liquor other than vodka and gin.

Middle-Glycemic Carbohydrates

• Oranges, peaches, plums, pears, and apples.

• High-protein pasta, yams, and Ezekial brand bread.

• Peas, pinto beans, kidney beans (canned), navy beans.

• Vodka and gin.

Low-Glycemic Carbohydrates

• Kidney beans, lentils, black-eyed peas, chickpeas, lima beans.

• Soya beans and soy products such as tofu, soy protein, tempeh, and miso. Be aware that soy products will often contain sugar.

• Nuts, milk, apricots, grapes, grapefruit, cherries, berries.

• Slow-cooked oatmeal and 100 percent whole-grain rye bread.

• Fructose and xylitol. These are the only low-glycemic sugars.

patients with diabetes, this means that almost all carbohydrates must be eliminated from the diet.

The Fat-Burning Factor

While the C-Factor is a specific indicator of how much your dietary carbohydrate intake is suppressing your fat metabolism, the Fat-Burning Factor evaluates conditions other than dietary carbohydrate that decrease your fat-burning potential. These other conditions include insulin resistance, hormonal deficiencies (particularly thyroid, cortisol, testosterone, and growth hormone), insufficient sleep, carnitine deficiency, coenzyme Q_{10} deficiency, dietary fat deficiencies, excessive trans-fatty acids, and vitamin and mineral deficiencies. The higher the Fat-Burning Factor, the more energy you are able to produce from fat. In fact, if you have an optimal Fat-Burning Factor, it can be taken as proof that you have none of the conditions given above.

The Fat-Burning Factor is determined by looking at the maximal amount of energy that your body is able to produce from fat during the exercise part of the test. The Fat-Burning Factor is a percentage calculation. It compares the expected or predicted fat-burning capability in a subject with what is actually measured from Bio-Energy Testing. In establishing the predicted values, the computer uses a default age of forty for subjects older than forty, and in overweight subjects the weight is corrected to an optimal body fat percentage. A Fat-Burning Factor greater than or equal to 100 is optimal because it indicates that your body is utilizing fat as an energy source with maximum efficiency. A value less than 100 indicates that any of the aforementioned conditions may be present.

People unable to lose weight often have a Fat-Burning Factor of less than 80 along with a C-Factor of less than 80. Functionally speaking, that means the majority of their daily energy needs are being met by carbohydrate metabolism. No wonder they can't lose weight. They can't burn fat! Only when the causes of their metabolic imbalances are corrected can they burn fat effectively and thus lose weight successfully.

This is of particular interest to a diabetic for two reasons. First, as I mentioned before, one of the principal factors in the development of diabetes is weight gain. Second, when the body can't burn fat well, cells have to rely more and more on glucose metabolism, which worsens blood sugar control and hastens the disease process. Thus, many cases of type 2 diabetes can be completely reversed simply by optimizing fat metabolism.

Optimal fat metabolism, as indicated by optimal C-Factor and Fat-Burning Factor, accomplishes a great number of other very desirable effects in addition to weight control, including:

• Decreasing your rate of aging

• Reducing the level of metabolic acids that contribute to chronic disease

• Increasing your endurance

• Increasing your energy levels

• Maintaining your blood sugar levels

• Lowering your cholesterol and triglycerides

Tiffany's Fat-Burning Factor was 74. You might wonder about how it is possible for fat burning to become so defective, but I can tell you that this score is not nearly as bad as I often see it. Many diabetics initially present with a Fat-Burning Factor of less than 50! As soon as I saw this value, I knew that it would be easier for her to reverse her diabetes.

The Fitness Factor

The Fitness Factor tells you how well the body is converting energy into power. It refers to the *maximum* total amount of power that the body is able to produce aerobically (from oxygen). The Fitness Factor is a function of energy production that takes into consideration overall strength, and as such, measures how well the muscles convert energy into power. It is determined by measuring the maximum amount of strength that you were able to demonstrate during the exercise part of the test. Fitness Factor is a percentage calculation. It compares the expected or predicted maximum strength in a subject with what is actually measured from Bio-Energy Testing. In establishing the predicted values, the computer uses a default age of forty for subjects older than forty, and in overweight subjects the weight is corrected to an optimal body fat percentage.

A low Fitness Factor—less than 100—is an indicator of one of the most common hallmarks of diabetes—a decrease in muscle mass, referred to as sarcopenia. Many doctors are aware that fat gain worsens diabetes, but very few understand that a loss of muscle mass is even more influential in this regard.

A Fitness Factor greater than or equal to 100 is optimal because it indicates that your body is preserving its muscle mass, and that you have not developed sarcopenia. Tiffany's Fitness Factor was 72, and although low, it's not all that bad. It indicated to me that once we implemented a program to increase her muscle mass, her diabetes would very quickly respond.

The Optimum Caloric Intake

It is currently well accepted by all diabetologists that obesity is critically important in diabetes. Simply correcting obesity in many cases has been found to completely eliminate the disease. The most common dietary cause of obesity is the excessive consumption of carbohydrates, particularly high-glycemic carbohydrates. Especially for diabetics, the secret to maintaining a healthy weight and controlling blood sugar is to limit eating high- and middle-glycemic foods, and in many cases, even the low-glycemic foods (see "The Glycemic Index" on page 29). However, another very common cause of obesity is just plain old overeating.

By overeating I am not talking about eating more than you see everyone else eating. The way I am using the word, overeating simply means taking in more calories than your particular metabolism is able to burn. In this day and age when meal portions are so large and high-calorie foods are so readily available, it is all too easy to overeat. Successful diabetes management often means monitoring your daily caloric intake.

The correct caloric intake for maximum advantage is very individual because it is a direct function of each individual's particular energy dynamics. Because it measures these dynamics, Bio-Energy Testing can determine the precise caloric intake needed to meet a particular individual's energy requirements with unprecedented precision. The Bio-Energy Testing analyzer is able to do this because it is measuring your energy production. Thus, since it knows how much energy you produce both when you are resting and when you are exerting, it can determine exactly how many calories your body needs to meet your energy needs.

Tiffany's optimum caloric intake, based on her actual levels of energy consumption, was 1,241 calories per day, which points out a very significant problem with predicted values for caloric needs. The problem is this: When I go to the physiology texts and look up the predicted caloric needs of a woman Tiffany's age and weight, I find the number is 2,300 calories. But this is more than 1,000 calories in excess of what she really needs!

Similar discrepancies show up with almost every patient I test, whether the patient is healthy or not and whether or not diabetes is present. It is important to know that these predicted values for caloric needs were first determined fifty years ago, and it may very likely be the case that in the last fifty years, metabolic rates, and subsequently caloric needs, have diminished.

Perhaps the decrease in caloric needs is due to increased levels of stress, lack of sleep, poor dietary habits, and/or some other modern-day phenomenon. Either that or the original measurements were not all that accurate. Whatever the reason, I can assure you that the predicted caloric needs that are routinely used to advise diabetics regarding their optimal caloric intakes are almost always excessive.

Only by using Bio-Energy Testing am I now able to accurately determine the correct caloric needs of my diabetic patients. Combined with correcting her fat metabolism, placing Tiffany on the appropriate amount of daily calories will be a critical factor in turning her case around.

The M-Factor (Metabolic Factor)

The M-Factor is a measurement of energy production at rest. It is a reflection of the overall metabolism of both glucose and fat when the subject is not exercising.

Just like with Heart Factor and Lung Factor, M-Factor is a percentage calculation. It compares the expected or predicted resting energy production in a subject with what is actually measured from Bio-Energy Testing. In establishing the predicted values, the computer uses a default age of forty for subjects older than forty, and in overweight subjects the weight is corrected to an optimal body fat percentage.

An optimal M-Factor is 100, indicating that the subject is producing optimal levels of energy while at rest. Low M-Factors are often associated with diabetes because low resting-energy production decreases insulin's ability to work and, therefore, increases insulin resistance. This is because insulin requires a substantial amount of energy in order to interact with the cell membrane and exert its effects.

Another very significant result of a low M-Factor is a decrease in the body's ability to release stored fat for energy production, which then forces the body to rely more on glucose metabolism. This is not a good scenario for a diabetic.

A low M-Factor can be caused by poor muscle mass, thyroid deficiency, adrenal insufficiency, excessive estrogen, progesterone deficiency, testosterone deficiency, growth hormone deficiency, dehydration, various nutritional deficiencies, and/or insufficient sleep.

A low M-Factor is the most sensitive indicator of low thyroid states, even when thyroid blood tests are in the so-called normal range. Tiffany's M-Factor was 83, indicating that her metabolism was running at about 83 percent of what would be optimal. This was not too surprising considering her overweight.

The EQ (Energy Quotient)

The EQ (energy quotient) is a measurement of the maximum amount of energy the body can produce aerobically, that is, from oxygen. Nothing is more tied to optimal mental and physical functioning and disease prevention than aerobic energy production.

In an impressive review article on the age-associated decline in aerobic capacity in men, the authors state, "Maximal aerobic capacity [that is, your EQ] is an independent risk factor for cardiovascular disease, cognitive dysfunction, and all cause mortality."[1] This statement is medicalese for "your EQ will single-handedly determine your risk of having heart disease, senility, and every known cause of death." This is particularly true for diabetics: since the very action of insulin on the cell membrane is dependent on energy production, each cell's sensitivity to insulin is a direct function of EQ

Your EQ is a global measurement that reflects the sum total of all the factors involved in energy production, including lifestyle, lung function, heart strength, circulation, fat metabolism, carbohydrate metabolism, toxicity, nutrient status, hormonal balance, liver and kidney function, fitness, and cellular bio-energetics. If any of these factors is less than optimal, it will result in a decreased EQ Thus, your EQ provides the definitive cross-check on all the physiological and biochemical functions required to prevent and treat diabetes.

The EQ is a percentage calculation determined by measuring your total aerobic energy production and then comparing it to what is predicted. In establishing the predicted values, the computer uses a default age of forty for subjects older than forty, and in overweight subjects the weight is corrected to an optimal body fat percentage.

An optimal EQ is 100 percent or greater, indicating that you are producing energy as well as you need to in order to stay healthy, reduce risk of disease, and slow down aging. Levels falling below 100 indicate the degree that illness, aging, and lifestyle factors are robbing you of a chance to improve and even cure your diabetes.

Tiffany's EQ was 91, not a bad EQ for a sixty-two-year-old diabetic, but still below what I felt was optimal for her. Her EQ indicated that improving her total effective energy production would substantially help her control her disease.

Biological Age—How Old Are You Really?

Alas, energy production steadily decreases with age. This decline results in diminished function in every single cell, tissue, and organ in the body. Decreased energy production is behind the symptoms and disabilities associated with diabetes, as well as the very process of aging itself. It is the single reason why type 2 diabetes is so closely linked to getting older.

The Bio-Energy Testing computer determines your biological age by matching your energy dynamics with persons of various ages. So basically, your biological age is the age at which your body is functioning.

If your biological age is less than your chronological age, congratulations! You have just cheated Mother Nature out of as many years. If your biological age is greater than your chronological age, you now know that you have some work to do to get back in line.

Remember that your chronological age only reflects how long you have been alive, and other than determining that you are going to have to spend more for life insurance and less at the movies, your chronological age is absolutely unimportant. It is your biological age—the age at which your body is functioning—that determines your health, your rate of aging, your resistance to disease, and your response to diabetes therapy. Like I always tell my patients, "No matter how many candles they stick in your birthday cake, your biological age is how old you *really* are!"

Tiffany's biological age was forty-eight years old. That means that despite her diabetic condition, her sixty-two-year-old body was still in the same working order as a woman's who was fourteen years younger. From this perspective alone, her prognosis looked very good, assuming she got her weight down and shifted her glucose-oriented metabolism back to fat.

The FBR (Fat-Burning Heart Rate)

Bio-Energy Testing is able to measure the level of energy that you are producing from fat while you are exercising. The fat-burning heart rate, or FBR, is the heart rate that you need to maintain while exercising in order to burn the maximum amount of fat possible. When you are exercising at your FBR, your body is burning fat as fast and as efficiently as it can.

As you exercise harder and drive your heart rate beyond your FBR, energy produced from fat metabolism progressively declines, while energy from glucose (sugar/carbohydrate) metabolism increases. This is because fat metabolism is not as fast as glucose metabolism, and also because glucose can produce more energy per molecule of oxygen than can fat. If you keep on steadily increasing your exercise intensity, you will get to a point at which you are not producing any energy at all from fat. At this point all energy production is coming from glucose.

Knowing your FBR is vitally important for diabetics because anything that maximizes fat metabolism will improve diabetes, and exercising at the FBR is exactly what does that. Additionally, when fat loss is an issue, it becomes important to spend a significant amount of your exercise time at your FBR.

As a general rule of thumb, I have found it important to make sure that my diabetic patients spend at least 80 percent of their exercise time at their FBR. Tiffany's FBR was 140 beats per minute, indicating that when she exercises at a level of intensity that causes her heart rate to be 140, her body is burning fat as efficiently as possible.

The ATR (Anaerobic Threshold Heart Rate)

Your ATR (anaerobic threshold heart rate) refers to the heart rate at which you are producing the maximum amount of energy that your body is able to produce from oxygen. This is the point of exercise I mentioned in the previous section, the point at which all of your energy production is coming from glucose and none from fat. When you are exercising hard enough to arrive at your ATR, you have reached your aerobic capacity, that is, the maximum amount of energy that you can get from oxygen metabolism. All energy produced when you are exercising above your ATR is produced without oxygen. This is called anaerobic energy production.

In order to feel the effects of anaerobic metabolism, simply hold your breath. After about one minute you will go into a state of 100 percent anaerobic metabolism. As you do this, you will start to experience the physical symptoms associated with anaerobic metabolism: breathlessness, dizziness, anxiety, panic, and pain. If you continue, you will eventually lose consciousness because anaerobic energy production is an extremely inefficient way to make energy.

Not only does anaerobic metabolism feel uncomfortable, it is as bad for you as it feels. It will take you less than a minute of holding your breath to figure out a few things about anaerobic metabolism:

- It can only meet your energy demands for a very limited amount of time. This is because the production of energy in the body from anaerobic metabolism is only a fraction of that produced when oxygen is used.

- The brain panics and eventually becomes nonfunctional. This is because the brain is the organ most sensitive to energy-deficiency states.

- It hurts! This is because anaerobic metabolism produces a huge amount of lactic acid, and excessive lactic acid causes pain in the muscles.

- You become breathless. This is because anaerobic metabolism causes a buildup of carbon dioxide, which is what drives your breathing rate.

Anaerobic energy production is undesirable for a number of other reasons as well. It causes accelerated aging by increasing irreversible free-radical injury to your RNA and DNA (your genetic material), exhausts your adrenal glands, which causes a host of medical conditions and symptoms, and creates elevated levels of acid in your tissues. This is why exercising above your ATR, the point where you enter into anaerobic energy production, for more than a few minutes is unhealthy for the general population, but is especially bad for diabetics.

These are important reasons why exercising above your ATR is *bad news*. Consider it like the red line on your car's RPM gauge. Your car can easily go over the red line, but you are damaging the engine when you do this because you are working it beyond its capability. Similarly, you are damaging the engines in your cells, the mitochondria, when you exercise above your ATR on any kind of regular basis.

However, it's an entirely different situation when you are exercising precisely at your ATR. In this case, you are training your body to produce energy at its maximum aerobic potential. This is the best way to achieve and maintain fitness.

I have found that diabetics typically respond best when they spend about 20 percent of their exercise time at their ATR. Tiffany's ATR was 150 beats per minute, indicating that she needs to make sure that when she is exercising she does not allow her heart rate to go above this number.

The Optimum Exercise Zone

Your optimum exercise zone is the heart-rate range bound on one end by your FBR and on the other end by your ATR. One of the beauties of Bio-Energy Testing is that we are able to determine your actual FBR and ATR, and therefore, your optimum exercise zone, instead of relying on a calculated formula. This turns out to be critically important because research (see Appendix B for information on my paper entitled "Is Your Patient Exercising Too Hard to Be Healthy?") has been able to demonstrate that calculated exercise formulas are almost *always* significantly inaccurate, and either result in patients exercising at dangerously elevated levels above their ATR or at inefficiently low levels below their FBR.

It is worthwhile to say it again: When you are exercising at too elevated a level of exercise for your physiology, your body will increase its level of free-radical damage. Your body, especially the islet cells of your pancreas, will actually wear out faster! Instead of reversing your diabetic condition, you will accelerate it.

Conversely, when you are exercising at too low a level of exercise for your physiology, your exercise will be inefficient, and you will be wasting valuable exercise time. So whenever you exercise, be sure to wear a heart-rate monitor, and be certain to keep within your zone. We will discuss exercise issues more in Chapter 8.

WHERE CAN MY ENERGY BE TESTED?

As of this writing, there are testing centers in Los Angeles; San Francisco; the Palm Springs area; Las Vegas; Portland, Oregon; Ashland, Oregon; Grand Junction, Colorado; Vancouver, Canada; and even as far away as Singapore. We are also preparing to install Bio-Energy Testing in hospitals that want to do more than just treat disease and are offering preventive medicine programs. To obtain the name of a facility in your area offering Bio-Energy Testing, visit the website www.bioenergytesting.com, or call toll-free 866-376-0610.

The cost for Bio-Energy Testing will vary depending on where you have it performed, but it typically runs in the area of $200 to $250. This is not a bad price for getting the kind of information that can turn your entire life around.

Now that you have a good working idea of how Bio-Energy Testing is performed and what the measurements mean, let's take a look at how I used this amazing technology to discover that type 2 diabetes is an energy deficit disorder.

CHAPTER 3

Diabetes Is an Energy Deficit Disorder

*"Of all the self-fulfilling prophecies in our culture,
the assumption that aging means decline and
poor health is probably the deadliest."*
—MARILYN FERGUSON, *THE AQUARIAN CONSPIRACY*

I coined the term "energy deficit disorder" in my first book, entitled *Bursting with Energy*. In that book, I proposed a new theory of aging that can also be applied to degenerative disease, including diabetes. The energy deficit theory of aging and disease is as follows:

1. The processes involved in aging and degenerative diseases are all energy dependent. They are caused and then accelerated by the following two interwoven conditions that act together to decrease energy production:

   • Suboptimal aerobic metabolism both at rest and during exercise

   • A shift away from a healthy state in which cells primarily use fat and protein for energy production to a pathological state in which cells primarily use glucose (sugar/carbohydrate) for energy production

2. The processes that lead to aging and degenerative diseases can be slowed down and even reversed by altering these two conditions and thereby increasing energy production.

An energy deficit disorder, therefore, is a disorder that results from a decrease in energy production stemming from the two conditions mentioned above. Let's begin with a look at the first condition.

SUBOPTIMAL AEROBIC METABOLISM

Everybody knows that not breathing is a sure way to have problems very quickly, but you may not have a good understanding of why that is. It's all about energy production. Your life utterly depends on a constant stream of energy production, so much so that as soon as that stream is interrupted even for one second, you will instantly die.

As mentioned, there are two ways your body can make energy. One way is by metabolizing the oxygen you breathe. This form of energy stems from what is called aerobic metabolism, and it is abundant and long lasting. The other way your body can make energy is from a process referred to as anaerobic (literally "without oxygen") metabolism.

Remember holding your breath? Anaerobic metabolism is a much less efficient form of energy production. This form of metabolism is only able to produce one-eighteenth as much energy as aerobic metabolism. In fact, it is only useful for emergencies because it is so inefficient that it can maintain life for a maximum of just three to five minutes.

Thus, clearly the most important way that your body can produce energy, and hence maintain life and optimal function, is by aerobic metabolism. To the degree that your body fails to adequately do this, it will be unable to produce enough energy. At this point, an energy deficit will result.

SHIFTING FROM FAT TO GLUCOSE

In order to understand the second condition, it will be necessary to describe how aerobic metabolism makes energy. There are two ways that your body can make energy aerobically. One way is to use oxygen to burn fat, and the other way is to use oxygen to burn glucose.

As you will see, despite the current wisdom of the day, which has been blindly accepted as a definite physiological principle, the facts show that fat, not glucose, metabolism is the primary way the body wants to make energy. This idea goes against the grain of everything the experts have told us for so many years. I discovered it quite by accident after I began using Bio-Energy Testing to determine the energy production of my patients.

Since fat and glucose are metabolized by oxygen in different ways, Bio-Energy Testing is capable of determining, amongst other things, whether the body is using oxygen to burn fat or to burn glucose. As I started testing patients, I gradually became aware of a certain pattern. The younger and healthier the patient was, the more he or she burned fat. In fact, the typical twenty-two-year-old athlete obtained almost 100 percent of his resting energy production by burning fat.

However, the older or sicker my patient was, the more energy he or she produced from glucose, instead of fat, metabolism. That same twenty-two-year-old, even if he continued to exercise and keep in shape, would be producing better than half of his resting energy from glucose by the time he reached fifty-five years old. I saw this extremely consistent shift from fat metabolism to glucose metabolism over and over again as people aged or developed illnesses.

I was busy wondering about this shift from fat to glucose metabolism when the following occurred to me: Why in the world would Mother Nature give us the capability of producing energy from two completely different sources? It makes about as much sense as having a car that has two fuel tanks, one for diesel and one for gasoline.

One thing I have learned over the course of more than thirty years of practicing medicine is that the body is not stupid. If it is doing something, it is doing it for a very good reason, and we should always heed its message. The only logical reason for two sources of energy is that each must be able to do certain things that the other is incapable of. So I began to study all the differences between fat and glucose as energy fuels.

You Can Store a Lot of Fat, but Only a Little Glucose

For one, the body has a large storage capacity for fat, whereas it has only a very minimal storage capacity for glucose. Just to give you an example of this difference, if your body was forced to live off only your glucose stores, you would die within only three to four hours. On the other hand, your body can store enough fat to last you for anywhere from weeks to months. Clearly, when analyzing storage capacity alone, it appears that Mother Nature meant fat to be the primary energy source, not glucose.

Glucose Is for Emergencies

There is another extremely important difference between glucose and fat metabolism that I have already alluded to. In the process of anaerobic metabolism, glucose (unlike fat) can be turned into energy even in the absence of oxygen. I asked myself why Nature would want us to have the capability to make energy without oxygen, and then the obvious occurred to me: glucose metabolism must have evolved for emergencies.

Say you were unable to breathe because of a fire or because you were drowning or being choked. If the only way you could produce energy were from fat, after the body's residual amount of oxygen in the blood was metabolized in thirty to sixty seconds, you would simply fall over dead. Thanks to glucose metabolism, that won't happen because your body can survive off glucose for an additional three to five minutes even in the absence of oxygen. This may not sound like much time, but it may be just enough time to help you get out of harm's way—just enough time for an emergency evacuation.

The other thing about glucose is that the body can make about 5 percent more energy from glucose per molecule of oxygen than it can from fat. This, in addition to the body's ability to make energy much faster from glucose than it can from fat, makes glucose much more suitable for emergencies. So, while Mother Nature designed fat to be the preferred source of energy 99 percent of the time, She developed the capability of glucose metabolism for urgent situations.

Why Fat at All?

So if glucose can provide more energy, and faster, than fat can, in addition to providing energy without depending on oxygen when fat requires oxygen, why in the world did Nature evolve fat metabolism? Why didn't we evolve with a mechanism to store large reserves of glucose and forget fat altogether? There are several possible answers to this question.

For one, fat can be stored much more efficiently than glucose because more than twice as many calories of energy can be stored per square inch as fat than as glucose. For example, a cup of butter holds more calories of energy than two cups of sugar.

Second, as our human physiology was initially evolving, food sources of fat were much more easily found than were glucose sources. Early humans fed primarily on fat and protein from killed animals simply because an animal food source that contains virtually no glucose was the only food source that was available throughout the year.

Don't forget that even though we live in a supermarket era, we still have caveman physiology, and when our physiology was evolving, I'm told, supermarkets were not around. Unless your ancestors lived in very temperate zones, they were unable to harvest any kind of fruit or vegetation for many months out of the year. So naturally they were forced to evolve a metabolism that thrived on animal fat and protein, and depended very little, if at all, on vegetation and fruit.

Glucose Makes More Acid

Lastly, there is one more difference between glucose and fat metabolism that results in fat having significantly more survival value than glucose, and that has to do with acid production.

One of those little physiological facts of life is that in order to make energy, our bodies must produce acid as a byproduct. Very basically, we produce energy by metabolizing a high-energy molecule called oxygen. It is in this process that energy is released and harvested by the body to generate life, and a byproduct of this process of energy production is carbon dioxide (CO_2).

You probably know all that, but what you may not know is that carbon dioxide acts as an acid in our bodies. Some people are erroneously of the opinion that so-called acid foods are responsible for the acid that accumulates in our bodies. But according to the physiology texts, carbon dioxide production generates more than 100 times more acid than these foods could possibly produce and is clearly much more repsonsible for acid accumulation than are acid foods.

The other really significant form of acid produced in the body is lactic acid, which is often formed in large amounts and, as you will see, is only associated with glucose metabolism. The point to remember here is that virtually all the acid that accumulates in our bodies comes from either lactic acid or carbon dioxide.

Now, when your body produces acid it has to remove it immediately through various chemical mechanisms, collectively referred to as acid buffering systems. These buffering systems are extremely important because acid will kill you rather quickly if it is not contained and removed.

Acid is a poison to our bodies, and in the presence of increased acid accumulation, all the organs and tissues become seriously damaged. An example of how acid can slowly destroy your body can be found in the all-too-common condition known as osteoporosis.

Osteoporosis results because calcium, which can buffer acid, is pulled from your bones to buffer and eliminate acid when your body becomes overly acidic. This turns out to be great for maintaining less acid in the body, but it is obviously bad for your bones, which will eventually wear out.

I'm just using your bones here as an example to make my point. You can be sure that the same kind of damage happens to all of your tissues and organs in the presence of too much accumulated acid.

Given this information, you will no doubt be interested to know that glucose metabolism results in a much higher production of acid than does fat metabolism. This is because glucose produces 30 percent more carbon dioxide and also significant amounts of lactic acid.

Fat, on the other hand, does not produce any lactic acid at all. Thus, a physiology that just burned glucose would have very little survival value because it would produce so much acid that it would very quickly burn itself out!

DIABETES AND ENERGY DEFICIT

So now you have a pretty good idea of what led me to postulate the energy deficit theory of aging and disease. Since every function of the human body, from DNA and tissue repair to immune system function, is entirely dependent on energy production, it seems reasonable to assume that the decrease in energy production that predictably occurs as we get older is likely to be the single most fundamental common cause for aging and the diseases of aging, such as diabetes.

Moreover, since energy production is almost exclusively a function of aerobic metabolism (that is, your EQ), anything that impairs aerobic metabolism will encourage disease and accelerate aging. On the other hand, anything that improves aerobic metabolism will prevent disease and slow down aging.

Furthermore, since the aerobic metabolism of fat, not glucose, is the most optimal form of energy production, anything that impairs fat metabolism will also impair energy production.

Diabetes is perhaps the single best example we have of an energy deficit disorder. Even in the stages leading up to diabetes, long before it actually develops, there are multiple signs of both a decrease in aerobic metabolism, and a shift away from fat metabolism to glucose metabolism.

How Decreased Aerobic Metabolism Results in Type 2 Diabetes

Our cells are analogous to batteries in the sense that they are used to store energy. Once they create energy from either fat or glucose, the cells are able to store the energy in a special molecule called ATP (adenosine triphosphate). The energy can stay stored in this molecule until it is needed.

Every single aspect of the functioning of our cells and organs is completely dependent on having an adequate amount of ATP present at all times. As you would expect, there are many control mechanisms to assure that as the cells use up their supply of ATP, more is immediately made. Thus, even while you are sleeping, or rather, *especially* while you are sleeping, your body continues to breathe and crank out vital amounts of ATP.

Most important among ATP's functions in the cells is to provide the energy for the interaction between insulin and the cell membrane. ATP's role here is critical because the cells of the body require insulin to take in glucose for energy production. In the absence of insulin, glucose cannot get into the cells and as a result rises up to very high levels in the bloodstream.

As you might remember from Chapter 1, the way insulin works is by forming an interaction with the cell membrane, the membrane that surrounds and contains the cell. It is this interaction that then allows glucose to enter through the cell membrane into the interior of the cell where it can be utilized for energy production.

The important point to make here is that this interaction between insulin and the cell membrane is entirely dependent on ATP. Therefore, as energy production decreases and the cell has less and less ATP, it will not be able to interact with insulin effectively. This is the condition known as insulin resistance, which I referred to earlier.

Now, I don't want to imply here that decreased energy production is the only cause of insulin resistance, because there are other factors that I will discuss later, but I do believe that it is the most important and the most pervasive factor. When the genes for diabetes are present, insulin resistance will surely lead to the disease unless it is corrected early enough. The most effective way to prevent it, and to correct it when it is present, is to optimize energy production.

Additionally, insulin resistance is not the only way that decreased energy production can cause diabetes. As you will see in Chapter 9, which details the importance of the liver, optimal liver function is critical to maintaining normal blood sugar control. But in order to do this, the liver requires enormous amounts of ATP. In fact, the liver has one of the largest requirements for ATP of any organ in the body. Thus, a decrease in energy production translates to a decrease in liver function and represents a step closer to diabetes.

Yet another way that decreased energy production can result in diabetes has to do with hormone production. One of the hormones in question is pretty obvious—insulin. In order for the pancreas to make insulin it must have plenty of ATP available on a regular basis. The more insulin that is required by the body, the more ATP the pancreas needs to make it.

As you will learn in later chapters, there are other hormones that are almost as critical for proper blood sugar control as insulin. Just like with insulin, the production of each of these hormones is dependent on an abundant supply of ATP.

Finally, the body needs ATP in order to protect the islet cells of the pancreas from the free-radical damage that leads to diabetes. As I mentioned in Chapter 1, the end result of insulin resistance is that the islet cells must make ever larger amounts of insulin to compensate for the fact that the cell membranes are not responding appropriately to the insulin. This is an important point to remember. As the islet cells are forced to do this, they become increasingly susceptible to damage from excessive exposure to the free radicals that are produced as a byproduct of insulin production.

These free radicals are so highly destructive that they eventually completely destroy the islet cells, and as a result, insulin levels drop and diabetes results. The important thing to know here is that the body has several enzyme systems that are able to protect the islet cells from this free-radical damage.

These enzymes are called antioxidant enzymes, and they are all dependent on ATP levels for both their creation and their maintenance. Thus, when there is not enough ATP because of decreased energy production, these protective systems are unable to adequately protect the islet cells from free-radical damage, and the development of diabetes is further encouraged.

How the Shift from Fat to Glucose Metabolism Results in Type 2 Diabetes

Fat is the preferred nutrient for aerobic metabolism. It has infinitely more storage capacity, burns more efficiently, and results in much less acid production. Young people who are healthy and fit have metabolisms that almost exclusively burn fat for energy. However, most people when tested thirty years later, because of the effects of excessive carbohydrate intake, stress, lack of exercise and sleep, and nutrient and hormone deficiencies, will have gone through an amazing change. Their metabolism will have shifted from primarily burning fat for energy to primarily burning glucose.

This fat-to-glucose shift then leads to a number of significant changes that, in the presence of the right genes, will cause type 2 diabetes. Here's how it works.

1. The shift from fat to glucose metabolism causes the cells of the body to burn more glucose. Because only tiny amounts of glucose can be stored, this results in a continuous depletion of glucose stores. This depletion, besides causing a decrease and unevenness in overall energy production, also forces you to eat more carbohydrate in order to replenish the stores.

2. The more carbohydrate you eat to replenish the stores, the more insulin your body will make to compensate for the increased intake. The cells of the body respond to this increase in insulin production by decreasing the amount of insulin receptors on their membranes. This process is called "receptor down regulation," and it leads to insulin resistance.

   Then, as we have already seen, in order to compensate for insulin resistance, your pancreas will make ever-increasing amounts of insulin. This vicious cycle, then, just intensifies over the years that follow.

3. Because you are eating more carbohydrate to replenish your continuously depleted glucose stores, your body will adapt to this dietary shift by focusing more and more on burning carbohydrate, and less and less on burning fat. Soon, as a consequence of this environment, it will begin to lose its fat-burning efficiency. Furthermore, since the majority of all those dietary carbohydrate calories are not going to be used immediately for energy production, they will be converted to stored fat.

4. Burning less and storing more fat leads to increases in your body fat percentage. Increased body fat causes insulin resistance, and as we have seen, the pancreas will then respond by making yet more insulin. Insulin is a potent blocker of fat metabolism, which then completes still another vicious cycle.

5. As your body is responding to each one of these consequences of the fat-to-glucose shift, the end result is always an increase in insulin levels. Since cortisol is the primary hormone your body uses to balance the effects of insulin, the increased insulin levels then cause your adrenal glands to compensate by increasing the production of cortisol.

6. Elevated cortisol levels are known to suppress the activity of the insulin receptors on the cells, and thus the emerging state of insulin resistance becomes even more pronounced.

7. Elevated cortisol levels also cause your body to convert your muscle tissue to glucose in order to maintain your new "addiction" to glucose. The subsequent breakdown and loss of muscle tissue from these excessive levels of cortisol is another cause of insulin resistance.

8. In order to compensate for the insulin resistance caused by all of the above factors, your pancreas is now finding itself forced to produce ever-increasing amounts of insulin. The islet cells of the pancreas will eventually burn out from free-radical damage, and diabetes will finally be diagnosed.

PUTTING IT ALL TOGETHER

I believe that understanding the two concepts of the energy deficit theory of disease, as elucidated in this chapter, is vital to having an understanding not only of how to treat diabetes more effectively but also, more importantly from my perspective, how to prevent it.

Therapeutic strategies need to be directed at increasing the overall aerobic production of energy, as is exemplified by an optimal M-Factor and EQ on Bio-Energy Testing, and reversing the shift from fat to glucose metabolism, as exemplified by an optimal C-Factor and Fat-Burning Factor. In the next chapter, I will review two different actual patient cases that will demonstrate what you have learned so far.

CHAPTER 4

On the Road to Diabetes

"Two roads diverged in a wood, and I—I took the one
less traveled by, and that has made all the difference."
—ROBERT FROST, POET (1874–1963)

iabetes doesn't just happen overnight. The twists and turns on the roads that ultimately lead to the diagnosis of diabetes take place over years, even decades. In this chapter I will reach into my files and present two real-life cases of patients of mine. Obviously, I have obscured any personal information that would lead to their identity, but in both cases, the facts are presented as they actually occurred.

In the first case, that of "Barbara," you will see what happens to a person who discovers early on that she is heading straight for diabetes and yet doesn't take the warning signs seriously, continuing to drive in the same direction at the same speed. Where she ends up is predictable.

The second patient is "Antonio." Antonio serves as an example of someone who had prediabetes like Barbara, but who took it to heart, made a U-turn, and completely turned around his medical future. His life is now entirely different, and his future is bright.

These patients are not unusual. In fact, they are very common examples of people I see every day. As has been mentioned before, diabetes is growing at epidemic rates, and will soon be occurring in just about every family in your neighborhood. The poor dietary, exercise, sleep, and other lifestyle habits that are so common in the American way of life are putting us on a fast track to diabetes. Unless you are busy doing something about it, diabetes is likely to come knocking on your door or the doors of your loved ones.

BARBARA'S STORY

Barbara is a fifty-four-year-old woman who is widowed, has two children, and has had a successful business career. When she first came to see me in 1997, she was currently looking to change the direction of her professional life. She had been working her regular job at a mortgage company, while at the same time attending school full-time, working toward a degree in psychology. She is a charming, energetic, enthusiastic, devoted, and giving person. I can't imagine anyone who wouldn't like Barbara.

At her first visit, Barbara reported that she had gained thirty pounds over the previous year "for no apparent reason," and was feeling tired and very low in energy. Although she was very enthusiastic about her life, she had a lot of anxiety about all the changes she was dealing with. The fact that she was also in the throes of menopause did not help that much either. When I asked her if there was any family history of diabetes, she responded that thankfully there was not.

Barbara was only getting four to five hours of sleep on average. She would stay up late at night to study, going to bed around midnight. About two or three hours after she fell asleep, she would wake up feeling wide awake, with thoughts of finances, her school, children, and other issues on her mind. She would then either get up and clean the house ("God knows it needed it") or read. Eventually she went back to bed, only to have to get up again in a few hours to start her day.

Her diet was fairly typical. She was on a high-carbohydrate, low-fat diet that at the time all the experts were telling her was so healthy for her. Like many of my patients, she just could not understand why she was gaining weight despite hardly ever eating any fat.

She had a cup of coffee with sugar in the morning, and for lunch a sandwich with some fruit and a Coke or another cup of coffee. For dinner she had a home-cooked high-carb meal followed by dessert. Oh and, yes, she was way too busy to exercise. "What are you crazy? I don't even have enough time to clean my house. How in the world can I exercise?"

As part of my comprehensive evaluation of Barbara, I ordered Bio-Energy Testing, a measure of her insulin level, a glucose tolerance test, and a hemoglobin A1c. You are already familiar with Bio-Energy Testing and insulin levels, so at this point, let me take a few moments to describe what the other tests are all about.

GLUCOSE TOLERANCE TEST

The glucose tolerance test is the single most sensitive way to diagnose diabetes. It is performed first thing in the morning. To prepare for it, the patient needs to have a decent night's sleep and refrain from eating and exercising on the morning of the test.

First, a blood sample is drawn and tested for its blood sugar, or glucose, level. Then the patient is given a sugar drink that tastes like soda pop. The drink contains a known amount of glucose, and the amount given is dependent on the patient's weight.

The drink will, of course, cause an immediate increase in blood sugar, which will then stimulate the body to produce enough insulin to control the rising sugar levels. After the drink is taken, blood sugar levels are drawn every half hour for two hours in order to see how well insulin is able to do its job. Levels higher than 200 milligrams per deciliter (mg/dl) indicate a diagnosis of diabetes. Levels between 140 and 200 indicate a condition known as glucose intolerance. Glucose intolerance is diagnostic of prediabetes.

HEMOGLOBIN A1c TEST

The hemoglobin A1c test simply involves one blood draw, which can be done without fasting and at any time of day. It evaluates the cumulative effect of blood sugar levels on the hemoglobin molecules in the red blood cells. How well your blood sugar levels are being controlled can then be determined by looking at how they are influencing your hemoglobin A1c.

Healthy blood sugar control is indicated by a hemoglobin A1c level of less than 5.5 percent. Higher levels indicate progressively decreasing blood sugar control. Greater than 6 percent is considered diagnostic of diabetes, and greater than 7 percent is considered to be an ominous sign because it indicates increasingly higher levels of blood sugar. Since red blood cells have a three-month life span, the hemoglobin A1c test gives an indication of how well your blood sugar has been controlled over the past three months.

While we were waiting for the tests to be performed and the results to come back, I told Barbara to decrease her intake of carbohydrates, counseled her about sleep and exercise, and gave her some vitamins and adrenal hormones to help her adrenal gland cope with all the stress in her life. I also told her that, for me, if it was a choice between a clean house and a healthy body, I would be more interested in the healthy body. At the same time, I also reminded her and myself that it was her body, her life, and her choice, not mine.

Barbara came back about two months later. She had not pursued any of the tests because "I just don't have the money right now," but she had decreased her carbohydrate intake. She had lost twelve pounds as a result, and was feeling pretty good about that. Furthermore, she reported that her energy level was much better as long as she remembered to take the adrenal hormones.

I saw her again after another two months, at which time she was continuing to feel good and had lost an additional eight pounds. Then, as often happens in this form of medicine, which involves lifestyle changes instead of just pills, Barbara stopped coming in, and I did not see her again until the year 2000.

THREE YEARS LATER

When Barbara came in this time, she reported that she had graduated from school and that her life was settling down somewhat. She also said that she now had the resources for the testing. She had been "sort of watching my diet," and her sleep was a little better. She was also occasionally exercising.

Her test results were not all that surprising. Her Bio-Energy Test revealed a low M-Factor, indicative of a low metabolism. Her C-Factor was extremely low, indicating that although she had decreased her carbohydrate intake, it was still way over the line.

Her Fat-Burning Factor was depressed, which just pointed to the obvious fact that she was not able to metabolize fat as well as she needed to. And her EQ was low, indicating a significant energy deficit state. We were seeing all the signs typical of the road to diabetes, decreased energy production along with decreased fat metabolism.

Not surprisingly, Barbara's insulin level was grossly elevated at 27 microunits per milliliter (mU/ml). This brings me to an important point, that of so-called normal laboratory levels.

Most laboratories report that the "normal" levels of insulin fall between 5 and 25 mU/ml. According to these standards, an insulin level must be greater than 25 mU/ml in order to be classified as abnormal, which Barbara's certainly was. However, in the great majority of cases any level over 10 mU/ml is indicative of insulin resistance.

The only reason laboratories report that values greater than 10 mU/ml are "normal" is because insulin resistance is a normal occurrence in the so-called healthy American population, which is used to determine what levels are acceptable and what levels are not. So even though laboratories report insulin levels as high as 25 mU/ml to be in the "normal range," any value greater than 10 mU/ml indicates a prediabetic state.

Barbara's blood lipids revealed the poor cholesterol ratio and the elevated triglycerides that are so common in both diabetes and the prediabetic state. The good news was that Barbara's hemoglobin A1c was below 6 percent, and her two-hour glucose tolerance test was 160 mg/dl, which meant that although she was definitely on the road to diabetes, she still had time to turn in another direction.

I counseled her to pretty much completely eliminate all carbohydrates from her diet, including high-, middle-, and low-glycemic carbohydrates (see "The Glycemic Index" on page 29). I started her on an herbal/nutrient combination designed to increase her body's sensitivity to insulin and also told her in no uncertain terms that she was heading in the wrong direction and that she needed to revamp her lifestyle. Besides needing to change her eating habits, she also needed to start getting to bed earlier.

Furthermore, now that the Bio-Energy Testing had provided her with the correct guidelines for her exercise program, she needed to really understand that living without regular exercise was going to keep her in jeopardy. So she was advised to treat herself to exercise at least thirty minutes out of every day of her life.

These directions constituted the map she needed to follow in order to end up where she wanted to be—that is, enjoying a life characterized by high energy, free from disease and discomfort.

Well, my little pep talk helped for a while, and she dropped an additional twenty pounds. More important, her insulin levels dropped to 14 mU/ml, and it was looking like she was responding to the changes she had made. Barbara's story, however, did not turn out nearly as well as I had hoped for her. After about three months she began to slip.

She became much less attentive to her body's needs and started slacking off a little on the diet and exercise program. Additionally, she still maintained her poor sleep habits. As a result, her follow-up blood work revealed that her insulin level had climbed again to 18 mU/ml, and her weight loss had come to an abrupt halt.

Because of these developments, I added the medication metformin, which is often very effective at increasing insulin sensitivity, to her program. With many people, taking a pill is a much more acceptable way to approach a problem than turning around their lifestyle.

EIGHTEEN MONTHS LATER

I scheduled Barbara to return for more follow-up testing in about six months, but I didn't hear from her until eighteen months later. When she called then, she was crying. "I stopped everything I was doing about a month after I last saw you except for the pills. It just seemed like it was too much for me. I have put all my weight back on plus an additional ten pounds. I feel lousy, and I was just told by another physician that I have diabetes. This terrifies me and I think I am ready now to do everything I can to change all this around."

Barbara now has diabetes, and so far we have not been able to reverse that. Fortunately, however, she finally came to grips with the facts of her life and made the necessary changes to bring her diabetes into complete control. Ironically, had she made these very same changes earlier, she would never have gotten diabetes in the first place.

ANTONIO'S STORY

Antonio was forty-three years old when he first came to see me back in the summer of 2001. He came complaining of the two symptoms that I hear the most in my practice, lack of energy and continuing weight gain.

At first I suspected that the majority of his problems stemmed from his occupation as a shift worker. My clinic is in Nevada, home of twenty-four-hour casinos, and I have a lot of patients who work during the night and sleep during the day. Inevitably, most of them fail to get enough sleep, because it's just plain hard to get adequate sleep during the day.

When I asked him specifically about sleep, he told me that on the five days per week that he works, he gets to bed around 6:00 A.M., and is usually able to sleep uninterruptedly for about six hours. This is hardly the perfect lifestyle, but I have other patients with sleep patterns that are much worse.

Antonio was very good about recognizing the importance of exercise; he was already spending forty-five to sixty minutes five days a week exercising. When I asked about a family history of diabetes, Antonio told me that his father and his grandfather on his father's side both had diabetes.

At a height of five feet, 10 inches, his weight was 280 pounds. Our body fat calculations determined that his ideal body weight was about 186 pounds. Either Antonio was 100 pounds overweight, or he was about three feet too short.

Virtually every one of his cholesterol and triglyceride numbers were dangerously high, and his glucose tolerance test was 155 mg/dl. This of course meant that he did not yet have diabetes but was moving in that direction.

His insulin level was quite elevated at 19 mU/ml. This was in the "normal" range, but, as I mentioned before, such a level is still indicative of insulin resistance and prediabetes. His hemoglobin A1c was 5.8 percent. This is still within the reference range but was a little over the 5.5 percent level that I consider to be optimal.

Antonio's Bio-Energy Testing was also revealing. His M-Factor equaled 79, indicating that his metabolism was about 79 percent of optimal. This not only is one of the reasons why he had been steadily gaining weight, but it was also an indicator of the early stages of decreased energy production.

His C-Factor, the indicator of whether or not he was eating too many carbohydrates for his physiology, was considerably low at 72. He thought that he was "being good" about his carbohydrate intake. Until he saw this value, he did not appreciate how carbohydrate intolerant he really was.

His Fat-Burning Factor was 58. This is particularly poor and indicated a severe problem with burning fat. No doubt his carbohydrate intake was one of the reasons for his decreased ability to burn fat, but at this level I was virtually assured that he additionally had some other abnormality of fat metabolism. His EQ was excellent, as would be expected because he was such a good exerciser. This was an excellent prognostic sign.

In short, all Antonio knew was that his energy was not quite as good as it should have been and that he had a real problem with his weight. What he did not know was that he was showing all the symptoms and signs of prediabetes, and that he was heading down the road to diabetes at a pretty good clip.

Antonio was one of those patients a doctor really loves working with. He had a genuine love of life and a strong desire to be healthy so he could continue to enjoy his life for as long as he could. He had seen what diabetes had done to his father and his grandfather and he wanted no part of it.

"Tell Me What to Do, and I'll Do It"

When I told Antonio about what we had found, he simply said, "Just tell me what to do, Doc, and I'll do it." Here's what we did.

He was given the thyroid hormones T3 and T4 in combination with the adrenal hormones cortisol and DHEA (dehydroepiandrosterone) to correct his low metabolism. He was also started on a program of herbs and nutrients that are known to enhance fat metabolism.

We then fine-tuned his exercise program. One of the real blessings about Bio-Energy Testing is that it has the capability of determining the optimum levels of exercise for each individual person. Not surprisingly, it turned out that Antonio was exercising at a pace that was too hard to be helpful for him. That's right, he was exercising too hard to be healthy. I touched on this interesting topic in Chapter 2 and will cover it in more depth in Chapter 8 (see also Appendix B).

We toned down his exercise level and tweaked it to his particular capabilities. He actually ended up exercising not only less intensely, but also for about half the time. I call it exercising smart instead of exercising hard.

Finally, I talked with Antonio about carbohydrates. I explained to him how he had been brainwashed into believing that carbohydrates were a necessary part of the human diet, and that it was quite possible for him to live the rest of his life in perfect health and never again eat carbohydrates. When you read Chapter 6 on diet, you will have a better understanding of exactly what I told him.

He decided to go along with the program and to avoid eating grains, fruits, root vegetables, legumes, and sweets, although he admitted that it would take some getting used to. After all, these foods made up more than half of what he had been eating his entire life.

After three months, Antonio returned for a follow-up visit. He had lost eighteen pounds and his energy levels were "unbelievably good." Antonio had been a really good customer. His insulin level had dropped all the way down to 6 mU/ml, a level I consider optimal. He no longer had prediabetes. In only three months, he had made a complete U-turn down the highway to diabetes, and was quickly heading in the other direction.

I no longer had to "sell" the program to Antonio. He was now a true believer. Not only that, he was excited about the fact that his exercise periods were so much more enjoyable ("I used to feel like I was killing myself"). Plus, he was really adapting well to his new diet: "It took me a while to get to this point, but now I not only have lost the weight, I have also lost my desire for those foods. I guess I realized that they were killing me, and they just didn't seem that attractive."

I hear words like these from every patient I see who has kicked a bad habit. Whether it be cigarettes, excessive alcohol, or any other undesirable lifestyle habit, when people learn how to live without it, the once insatiable desire for it becomes very manageable. It just seems like you have to get over that initial hump of resistance. Antonio had gotten over that hump so far, and now all he had to do was keep going in the direction he was headed and not get sidetracked.

The Happy Ending

It's now been four years since I first met Antonio. I just saw him in the clinic the other day for his routine checkup. I'm sure that the reason I decided to include his case in this chapter is that he is so fresh on my mind, and he has continued to do so well.

His insulin level continues to be optimal at 6.6 mU/ml. His cholesterol and triglyceride levels as well as his hemoglobin A1c are all also optimal. He now weighs 185 pounds and has been easily maintaining this weight for the past eight months. He feels like a million bucks, and his Bio Energy Testing results are perfect. He continues to avoid carbohydrates "like the plague," and has happily adjusted to his new lifestyle. And as long as he remains true to his course, he will never ever have to hear some doctor say, "I'm sorry to have to give this news to you, Antonio, but you have developed diabetes."

I shared with him that although I have been fortunate enough not to have been born with his fat-sparing genes, I also pretty much avoid the carbs as much as he does, just because I have seen how detrimental they can be. We both agreed that living a healthy lifestyle may take a little getting used to at first, but it becomes second nature after a while, and the energy we feel along with the excellent quality of life is easily worth it.

READING THE SIGNS ALONG THE WAY

Are you on the road to diabetes? As the two cases described above illustrate, unless you know the signs, it is all too easy to be far along the way and not even realize it. The earlier you know about a prediabetes or diabetes condition, the easier and more effective will be the treatments. Here are the key questions to ask yourself:

- Is there a family history of diabetes?

- Are you over forty years old?

- Are you experiencing low energy levels?

- Are you having trouble with your weight?

- Are you getting less than eight hours of sleep per night?

- Are you experiencing too much stress?

- Do you not exercise regularly?

- Do carbohydrates make up more than 40 percent of your diet?

- Do you crave carbohydrates?

- Do you find it impossible to not eat carbohydrates?

- Do you have low levels of stamina?

- Are you out of shape?

No matter what your age, if you answer yes to any of the above questions, you should have the following tests done. These tests will help identify any tendency you have to either diabetes or prediabetes long before either of them become manifest:

- Bio-Energy Testing—Strong indicators that you are on the road to diabetes are a decrease in energy production, as manifested by a suboptimal M-Factor and/or EQ, and a decrease in fat metabolism, as is shown by a low C-Factor and a low Fat-Burning Factor.

- Cholesterol—A low HDL (good) cholesterol and an elevated LDL (bad) cholesterol are signs that you may have or may soon develop diabetes or prediabetes.

- Triglyceride levels—The so-called normal level is up to 180 mg/dl (milligrams per deciliter), but optimal levels are below 100.

- Hemoglobin A1c level—This should be below 5.5 percent.

- Fasting insulin level—This should be below 10 mU/ml. The optimal level is close to 5 mU/ml.

- If you are already taking insulin, the best way to follow how much insulin your body is making is to check your C-peptide levels. If your levels are greater than one nanogram per milliliter (ng/ml), it is possible that you will no longer require taking insulin if you work with a physician who closely follows the guidelines in this book.

- Two-hour glucose tolerance test—At no time should the glucose level go over 140 mg/dl.

If you are over the age of forty, you are at risk for developing diabetes — regardless of whether or not you answer yes to any of the above questions, or whether you have a family history of diabetes. You should have the above tests performed, along with the following additional tests, at least once every five years:

- A thyroid hormone assay: free T3, free T4, TSH.

- An adrenal hormone assay: fasting cortisol, DHEA.

- A sex hormone assay: testosterone, dihydrotestosterone, and estradiol for men; estrone, estradiol, estriol, testosterone, and progesterone for women.

- A growth hormone assay: twenty-four-hour urine for growth hormone, IGF-1.

I will be discussing these additional tests and their implications for the prevention and treatment of diabetes in the chapters to come.

The two real-life stories presented in this chapter are just a sampling of similar cases occurring all over the world right now. They serve to vividly portray how important it is to diagnose prediabetes, and just how effective simple lifestyle and nutritional therapies can be in preventing this disease. They also serve to illustrate how denial, procrastination, and lack of self-discipline can sabotage even the best of intentions.

According to the American Diabetes Association, in 2002 medical bills for diabetes cost the nation close to $92 billion! This almost doubled the amount spent in 1997. If loss of productivity is factored in, the cost of diabetes rises to $132 billion. What we will be paying in ten years is simply beyond comprehension. But that's just the monetary cost.

The real cost of diabetes is immeasurable, because it kills 180,000 people each year, and is the leading cause of blindness, kidney failure, limb amputations, and heart disease. We could engage in several full-scale wars at the same time, and it would still cost us less than what we already pay in death, suffering, and dollars for diabetes. All this for a problem that is completely preventable for pennies a day!

It's All About Energy— Eight Steps to Success

CHAPTER 5

Making the Change

*Understand that the right to choose your own path
is a sacred privilege. Use it. Dwell in possibility.*
—OPRAH WINFREY, ACTRESS AND TELEVISION TALK-SHOW HOST

A s I started off saying in the first part of this book, diabetes is an energy deficit disorder. Treating it, then, is "all about energy." Here in Part II, I will discuss eight crucial ways you can prevent diabetes and also dramatically improve your blood sugar control. These steps are all natural and easy, and most of them won't cost you a thing—they are simply lifestyle changes.

What these eight steps or changes have in common is a focus on the two core processes that cause diabetes in the first place:

1. They increase energy production by increasing oxygen metabolism.

2. They bring about a shift in energy production away from glucose metabolism and toward fat metabolism.

First of all, make it a point to find a Bio-Energy Testing facility and have your energy-production capabilities thoroughly analyzed. To find a testing center in your area, visit the website www.bioenergytesting.com. This amazing technology is invaluable in many ways, as discussed in Part I, and it will also connect you with a physician who is familiar with the concept of diabetes as an energy deficit disorder. If you have to travel to have the test performed, it will be well worth it. I have patients from as far away as Italy come to my clinic once a year just to have themselves tested and their program reevaluated.

The treatments are easy—it's the change in lifestyle that can be hard. But change is always hard, nothing new about that. Here are a few pointers about change in general that I have found to be very helpful to my patients over the years.

First, make sure that you remain at all times aware not only of why you are making the change, but also of how and why you will benefit from the change. Keep the intensity of your focus on a vision of yourself healthy, energetic, and free of the effects of diabetes for as long as you live. See the positivity of your choice, and remember that although you are losing your doughnuts, and so on, you are gaining something much more valuable—your life.

Next, give yourself time to adapt to the changes. It is not in your interest, or in the interest of the program, to become stressed out by the process of establishing a healthier lifestyle and getting control of your diabetes. I don't want you to feel overwhelmed. Don't rush out and try to do everything at once. Take my recommendations and then carefully apply them in a sequential manner.

Start with the diet, because that is usually the hardest for my patients to accept, and it shows huge and immediate rewards. After that, work on the supplements. This will be easier. It's always easier to take a pill, or in this case many pills. Once you have made these two changes, then incorporate the exercise, and you will be basically over the hump. Also, depending on your age and your particular condition, it may not be necessary to incorporate every single step. For example, if stress or lack of sleep do not play much of a role in your life, then the steps involving these topics can be skipped.

CHANGE IS HARD—AT FIRST

Change is hard. Routine is easy. Remember that the first few weeks of making any change are always the hardest. However, once the changes have become a part of your everyday life, they, too, will become routine and automatic. You can count on feeling some resistance at first, but I promise you that this resistance will dramatically decrease over the first eight weeks. I can't tell you how many patients I have treated over the years who have repeatedly told me, "Doctor, I just can't do that. I love my _____ (cigarettes, sweets, bread, whatever) too much," only to tell me six months later, "If I never have that again it will be just fine. I never thought I would feel this way about it."

I know of very few people who started walking immediately after they first stood up and never fell again. Falling didn't stop you when you were learning to walk, and it won't stop you now. If you stumble and break with your program, you may hear a little voice telling you, "See, I told you so. I knew you couldn't do it. It's no use. You might as well give up because you're never going to be successful with this crazy idea of yours." Listen to it and then ignore it, get up, and start walking again. Failures are simply steps along the way to success.

ENLIST SOME HELP

Get some help. How many successful athletes do you know who never had a coach to inspire them and kick them in the pants when they needed it? You will certainly need a doctor who has an understanding of what you want to do and achieve, and it may take some persistence to find such a physician. Not all doctors will be helpful in this regard. Appendix A lists some websites to help you find a suitable doctor.

Also, consider working with a fitness trainer for exercise and a nutritionist to help you with the diet changes. You may also find that cooking classes are just as helpful as they are fun.

"YOU DON'T UNDERSTAND. I CAN'T STOP."

I had a sixty-six-year-old patient named Johnny who worked for the railroad. Not only did his train smoke, but he did too—four packs of Lucky Strikes a day. Although I asked him many times to stop, and warned him of all the dangers that he already knew about anyway, he always told me, "You young guys just don't get the nature of addictions. You don't understand. I can't stop. Even if I wanted to, I can't stop."

Well, guess what. About three years later, Johnny started coughing up blood, and while he was in the hospital having his diagnostic tests done, he had to stop smoking. Somehow he didn't seem to mind. He was too concerned about the strong possibility of finding out that he had cancer.

Well, the tests came back indicating that he simply had a case of bronchitis. There was no cancer at all! That wake-up call inspired Johnny so much that from that day forward, he never had another cigarette.

Of course I used every opportunity I had to tease him about how it was really he who didn't get the nature of addictions. When the motivation is strong enough, addictions take a back seat. If you want to be healthy badly enough, you can do whatever it takes. That's just human nature.

I often hear: "Why should I change my lifestyle? I have diabetes in my genes, and there's no changing my genes"; "I'm going to get it anyway, so I might as well wait until I get it and then just take the drugs and do the best I can with it"; or, "My doctor told me that I was going to have diabetes forever, and that there was no chance of changing that. He also said that there is nothing other than medications to help with the problem." I hope this book has already convinced you that genetics play a relatively small role in whether or not most people get diabetes and in how well it can be controlled.

Follow these eight steps and you will be like many of my patients who have surprised not only themselves but their doctors as well. Now let's get started.

CHAPTER 6

STEP ONE:
Diet

To lengthen thy life,
lessen thy meals.

—BENJAMIN FRANKLIN, AUTHOR,
DIPLOMAT, INVENTOR, PHYSICIST,
POLITICIAN, AND PRINTER (1706–1790)

Although sleep and exercise are extremely important for the prevention and treatment of diabetes, there is nothing as important as learning to eat correctly. Unfortunately, we live in a society that has taught us and continues to encourage us to eat in such a way as to utterly guarantee malnutrition.

When I was in Singapore recently, some of my Singaporean friends introduced me to a delicacy there, a fruit by the name of durian. To them this "fabulous-tasting" fruit was a real treat, but to an outsider such as myself the smell and taste were absolutely disgusting. My friends were kidding me by calling it an acquired taste, and said that Asians have the same response to blue cheese. I could understand the comparison because I love blue cheese. It just reminded me of how strong our cultural experience is in determining what we think tastes good.

If you want to eat well and healthfully, you will have to get used to bucking your culture. Many of your friends will think that you have turned into a health nut, or that you have been indoctrinated by some kind of food cult. Please don't let any of these considerations affect you. Just do what's right, even if the rest of the neighborhood is sucking down convenience foods and carbohydrates like they are about to go out of style because they "taste so good."

ESSENTIAL CARBOHYDRATES?

There are three macronutrients: carbohydrate, fat, and protein. All foods can be analyzed in terms of just these three components.

As you will read in this chapter, there are eight essential amino acids (the components of proteins). "Essential" nutrients are essential to life. If you don't take them in in optimal amounts, you will develop various diseases or, in some cases, even die.

There are two essential fats that you will also read about. Again, the designation "essential" means that your very life and state of health depend on getting enough of these fats through your diet.

The point I want to make here is that there are *absolutely no* essential carbohydrates. Yes, that's right. You could go through your entire life without ever eating a carbohydrate and be perfectly healthy. In fact, you would be a lot healthier than if you were to eat anywhere close to the amount of carbohydrates commonly eaten in today's modern world. The only value at all to foods high in carbohydrates is their fiber and their nutrient content, and both of these can be more easily found in vegetables, which have an almost negligible amount of carbohydrate.

This might be a good time to clarify the difference between carbohydrate, as I use the word in this book, and fiber. It is true that technically speaking fiber is classified as a carbohydrate, but unlike all other carbohydrates, it is not absorbed and turned into glucose. Thus, it does not cause the rise in blood sugar that is so commonly seen with every other carbohydrate, and it does not need to be avoided. In fact, many studies have shown that diets high in fiber are beneficial in many ways.

Additionally, the fiber that is often quoted as being so abundant in high-carbohydrate foods such as grains is for the most part "insoluble fiber." Insoluble fiber is beneficial for bowel regularity, but other than that has virtually none of the detoxifying and healthy intestinal effects that are found in "soluble fiber." Unlike grains, the fiber found in vegetables is almost exclusively of the soluble kind.

So as long as you are eating enough vegetables, you are getting plenty of the healthy fiber that your body requires, and there is no need at all to add any carbohydrate to your diet. I place all high-carbohydrate foods in the same category as chocolate cake. They taste good and they're fun to eat, but they need to be avoided by diabetics because, like chocolate cake, they offer nothing nutritionally that can't be had from low-carbohydrate foods. Furthermore, high-carbohydrate foods have profound negative effects on both total energy production and fat metabolism.

Using Bio-Energy Testing, I have encountered many young, otherwise healthy thirty- to forty-year-old men and women whose high-carbohydrate diet has caused them to have ominously low energy-production numbers more typical of their grandparents. Were these people left to their own dietary devices, there is no doubt that in another ten to twenty years, many of them would have developed diabetes, cancer, or heart disease as a result of their poor food choices. The rewarding part has been that retesting such individuals after only three months of being off carbohydrates consistently reveals their energy production to have returned to optimal levels for their age.

So someone such as myself who does not have diabetes should only have carbohydrates as a "treat" and should not consider them worthy of being a regular part of the diet. From a dietary perspective, there is nothing more damaging to your health than the overingestion of carbohydrates, and the only thing essential about them is that they are essentially unhealthy and ought to be essentially avoided.

You Don't Mean . . . You Do?

So what exactly am I referring to when I use the word "carbohydrate"? Well, think of many of your favorite things to eat and you won't be too far off. See the glycemic index on page 29 for a list of the carbohydrate foods I'm talking about.

Of course, the worst carbohydrates are the sugars. Basically, anything that tastes sweet is a sugar unless it was sweetened with an artificial sweetener or a sweet herb such as stevia. For the most part, even if the label tells you it is sweetened with a "natural sugar," if it tastes sweet, it's a sugar and should be avoided. There are, however, two notable exceptions to this rule: xylitol, which comes from plums and raspberries, and fructose. The molecular makeup of these sugars gives them the unique property of being sweet, while at the same time having very few of the negative effects common to carbohydrates, and they can be used *in moderation* when you just "need" to have something sweet.

Next, almost as bad a choice as the sugars are the grains and anything that comes from grains. This includes wheat, corn, oats, barley, rye, rice, quinoa, and so on. It also includes flours made from these grains. This means bread, rolls, pasta, chips, hot cereals, cold cereals, and so on. I told you carbohydrates were going to be some of your favorite foods.

Other carbohydrates that need to be shunned are the root starches, or tubers. This category includes almost all of the foods that grow under the ground, such as potatoes, yams, carrots, sweet potatoes, beets, cassava and yucca (not to mention the starch gotten from these vegetables, tapioca, which is so commonly used), and so on. Fortunately, onions and garlic are not a problem—you can have as much of them as you want. But stay away from the rest.

Legumes (pod foods such as beans and peas) are a fabulous source of fiber and protein, but unfortunately they also contain a large amount of carbohydrate. Of all the carbohydrates, they are the best dietary choices for the nondiabetic. Depending on the severity of a given case, they can be eaten occasionally by diabetics.

Finally, there are the fruits. Fruits of any kind, including fruit juice, are a well-known recipe for disaster for diabetics, and they need to be avoided along with all of the other carbohydrates mentioned above.

FATS

Nearly your whole life, our culture has been telling you that fats are bad for you. Whenever I start discussing diet with patients, the first thing out of their mouths is that they are really trying to cut down on the fat.

What a great brainwashing the food industry has accomplished! Almost everybody thinks of fat as something to be avoided like the plague. The majority of the population, even many "experts," has been long convinced that for the sake of health, we should invest our food dollars in industrially altered food that has had the fat removed.

"Fat's the enemy," we are repeatedly told. And, like the cavalry, the food manufacturers are riding to our rescue with low-fat and nonfat substitutes to protect our health and correct the mistakes of Nature. I used to buy into this nonsense as well. Years ago I also believed that dietary fat raised blood fats and created atherosclerosis, hypertension, and heart disease. I was convinced that dietary fat was the cause of obesity. I even remember one expert who wrote that dietary fat caused diabetes.

I began putting all my diabetic patients on low-fat programs. Guess what happened? Nothing! Almost nobody lost weight. Blood sugar control didn't improve, and my patients continued to complain of fatigue, depressed immunity, insomnia, and so forth. In fact, they were beginning to resent me for putting them on a program that was extremely difficult to follow and did not taste good. Regardless of studies and what experts say, there is really no better litmus test than patient feedback. Patients live in the real world, not in laboratory cages.

Low-Fat Diets = Low-Energy Diets

The lack of results and the negative reactions I found with low-fat diets caused me to do a lot of rethinking. I was indeed "practicing" medicine by placing my patients on an abnormal diet. The human body did not evolve on a low-fat diet. Anthropological studies overwhelmingly concur that the original human diet was filled with meat *and* fat. Studies of the Eskimos and the Masai, whose traditional diets consist of virtually nothing but meat and fat, revealed a complete absence of heart disease, hypertension, and diabetes. It was only when they "modernized" and began eating flour and sugar that they developed these diseases.

I began thinking about the diets patients had when they first came to me. I asked myself how many diabetic patients ate a diet high in fat? I checked the dietary records. The answer was none. How many of my patients with heart disease actually ate a diet high in fat? None. How many of my patients with eating disorders gorged themselves on fat? None. Why not? The answer came to me rather quickly when I finally asked the question. People do not develop diseases or obesity from eating too much fat. It can't be done. You can't eat too much fat even if you try.

I once experimented on myself. I broiled a well-marbled steak, then covered it with butter. I ate slowly and quickly discovered that I was stuffed before I had even finished one-third of it. Compared with carbohydrate, fat and protein sit very long in the stomach in order to be digested. So you feel full. For most people, if they eat slowly enough and if they make sure not to gorge themselves, it is almost impossible to overeat on a diet high in meat and fat. Blood sugar actually stabilizes, and many disorders of the stomach and bowels improve.

Fat is not only the most preferred, most available, and most basic food source of energy. It is so much more. Unlike carbohydrate, which doesn't contribute anything to the structure and composition of the body, fat, along with protein, is what your body is made of. It is definitely *not* something to be avoided.

All of our cell membranes are made from fat. And over half the energy our cells produce goes into maintaining the integrity of these membranes. Research has shown that the very first pathological findings, when cells become diseased or poisoned, occur in the membranes. Without healthy membranes, the ability of the cell to create energy is severely impaired.

Your nervous system and your brain are almost completely made up of fats. Fats also serve as the building blocks for the steroid hormones, including cortisol, DHEA, and all the sex hormones. Fats make up prostaglandins, compounds that are intricately involved in the function of the immune system, the cardiovascular system, and the healing process after injury.

In this light, we can understand why Mother Nature gave us fat to eat. And why fats should be appreciated and not avoided. Without an adequate supply of fat, we could not even begin to maintain our mental and physical health.

Types of Fats

There are three categories of dietary fat: saturated, unsaturated, and monounsaturated.

Saturated fat turns solid in temperatures less than 70°F. Although saturated fats have been blamed for every health disorder from acne to cancer, they are actually a very healthy source of energy substrate and fat-soluble vitamins. The truth is that saturated fats only become a problem when they are eaten in excess and, as a result, edge out other foods such as protein sources and vegetables. Unfortunately, it is fairly easy to have an excessive amount of saturated fat in your diet if you eat meats, eggs, and dairy products that come from grain-fed animals, because grain-fed animals have a much higher percentage of fat per gram of protein. This is another one of our marvels of modern-day living. All of our meats, dairy, and eggs now come from grain-fed animals. The reason? Grain has the same effect on animals that it does on humans. It fattens them up. That makes the animals better for the market and the humans better for the medical industry.

On the other hand, animals fed on vegetables or grass instead of grain have a remarkably different fat makeup. They have significantly less saturated fat and more of what is called omega-3 unsaturated fat. Unsaturated fats, unlike the saturated kind, remain liquid (unless they have been hydrogenated) at room temperature. Omega-3 fats are one of the two essential fats that you need in your diet. They occur in non-grain-fed animals such as fish and shellfish, and are also found in vegetables and flaxseeds. You will hear more about omega-3 fats in a moment.

The other essential fat is called omega-6 fat, which is predominantly found in grains and seeds. Both omega-6 and omega-3 fats are unsaturated and essential. They must be found in optimal amounts in your diet in order for you to survive and maximize your health.

The third category is monounsaturated fats. These fats are like saturated fats in that they are not essential, but they are effectively used by the body for an energy source. Olive oil and coconut oil are examples of monounsaturated fats.

Not All Fats Are Created Equal

Nature indeed has given us fat to eat. So, too, has man. And it is with the manmade fats that the problems start. Take one guess as to which fats lead to immune suppression, heart disease, diabetes, macular degeneration, arthritis, hormonal deficiencies, and premature aging. And now, take a guess at which fats the food industry has been pushing.

Decades ago, food manufacturers encountered a problem transporting and storing processed "foods" (I use quotation marks because these so-called foods are more like garbage than food): the unsaturated fats in their products quickly became rancid. In order to make their merchandise more widely available, the industry had to surmount the rancidity issue.

Food scientists provided the answer: technology known as "hydrogenation" and "partial hydrogenation." These methods alter naturally occurring fats in such a way that they do not become rancid. Moreover, these new fats are so foreign to Nature that even bacteria and insects cannot survive on them. The ideal commercial fat was created—a fat that could be stored for years without rancidity or attack from Nature's predators.

Man had finally "improved" on the old-fashioned natural fats. Now we had margarine. It could sit on the countertop and thumb its nose all day, in fact for months on end, at rancidity. Man could now have a cornucopia of new "foods" with long shelf lives by using hydrogenated and partially hydrogenated fat technology in breads, mayonnaise, peanut butter, breakfast cereals, and so on, ad infinitum.

The only problem with the breakthrough is that these synthetic fats are alien to the body. They can't perform all the essential functions that natural omega-3 and omega-6 fats can. Worse yet, they actually act to interfere with the function of these natural fats. In fact, several published studies have documented that these hydrogenated fats, which are found in virtually every form of processed food, are able to block the ability of your mitochondria to produce energy.

Furthermore, they don't maintain adequate cell membrane potentials. They adversely affect the cell membrane receptors that are basic to hormone function. They block the activity of the enzyme plasmin that dissolves platelet clots. This effect increases the risk of developing blood clots that can cause life-threatening heart attacks.

Recent publications have also demonstrated that hydrogenated fats actually damage the inner walls of the arteries, thus contributing to cardiovascular disease. Researchers have documented that the increased consumption of margarine exactly parallels the modern-day epidemic of heart disease. Other studies have shown that manmade fats change the composition of the cell membranes in the heart, and that these changes are associated with heart disease.

A Question of Balance

So, omega-3 and omega-6 fats are the ones that are essential to your health. They are destroyed by the process of hydrogenation, and not only that, ingesting them after they have been hydrogenated will also impair energy production. But that's not the whole story. There is also a question of balance that is very important, particularly to people with diabetes or those on the road to diabetes.

Omega-3 and omega-6 fats perform different functions. Omega-6 fats act to increase inflammation and make your blood clot, whereas omega-3 fats do just the opposite. Both of these functions are essential to your health. Inflammation is the primary method your body uses to heal itself and protect itself from infections, pollutants, and cancer, and if your blood did not have the capability of clotting, you would very quickly bleed to death.

The problem is that our modern-day diets consist of an overabundance of omega-6 fats compared with omega-3 fats, and this imbalance skews our health in the direction of inflammation and thick or sticky blood. Let me just quote from a 2004 article, entitled "Omega-3: The Vanishing Nutrient Beyond Cardiovascular Prevention and Treatment," which in many ways sums up this imbalance issue. The authors state, "Omega-3 appears to be an important nutrient component of the mammalian body; however because of changes in the food chain during the last century it has become increasingly rare in frequently eaten foods. Currently, the main source of omega-3 is fish, which tends to be expensive and is periodically found to be contaminated. Common foods such as eggs, chicken, etc., which were once a rich source of omega-3, are now lacking it. Given the importance of omega-3 in a variety of body functions, as well as in the prevention of disease, it is obvious that in the coming years the scientific community worldwide will have to target agricultural research and development to the enrichment of foods with omega-3."[1] The "changes in the food chain" the authors are referring to is the switch from feeding animals vegetables and grass to feeding them grains.

This imbalance in fats has been cited as a significant factor in the development of cardiovascular disease, hypertension, cancer, and, yes, diabetes. To quote an article that appeared in the journal *Diabetes Research* that examined the use of 3 grams of omega-3 oils per day, "In type 2 diabetes dietary supplementation of omega 3 fatty acids improves insulin sensitivity and lowers plasma triglyceride levels."[2]

Also, it must be mentioned that some studies have shown that excessive doses (8 grams per day or more) of omega-3 oils may actually increase fasting blood sugar by as much as 20 percent. Apparently, these doses may push blood sugar levels of some patients too far in the wrong direction.

The bottom line on fats: don't be nearly so concerned about how much fat you eat as about what fat you eat. It's a good idea to avoid eating grain-fed meats as much as possible. Fish, shellfish, and lamb are usually not grain-fed, and grain-free beef and eggs are starting to become commercially available.

Avoid using omega-6 oils such as corn oil and safflower oil, and instead cook with olive oil. Being a monounsaturated oil, olive oil will not upset the omega-3/omega-6 balance.

And by all means, avoid hydrogenated and partially hydrogenated foods like the plague. Read the labels and you will find these oils in almost every product on the market.

High Fat and Low Fiber

What about medical reports showing an increase in cancer among people who eat high-fat diets? First, let me say that many of these studies are seriously flawed. Total caloric intake and incidence of obesity are almost never taken into account. The numbers of people monitored in these studies are relatively small, and the supposed increase in cancer is modest at best. Moreover, there are many contradicting studies.

For example, breast cancer is often said to be strongly associated with excessive dietary fat. In a long-term study monitoring the health and habits of 90,000 nurses, some 601 cases of breast cancer developed. However, there was no evidence of any relationship to fat intake.[3]

In another study, published in the *Journal of the National Cancer Institute*, researchers pointed out that while obesity and excess calorie intake have been implicated in cancer in both human and animal studies, fat intake per se has not. In this study, rats were exposed to a breast-cancer-causing agent and then fed a diet high in fat but restricted in calories, or a diet low in fat but with a much higher level of calories in the form of carbohydrate. Only 7 percent of the rats on the high-fat diet developed breast cancer, compared with 43 percent of those on the low-fat, high-calorie (high-carbohydrate) diet.[4]

Countering the supposed dietary-fat connection, a review of the medical literature reveals many impressive studies linking deficiencies of fiber, vitamins, and other nutrients to cancer. I believe that any possible fat connection can be explained by the fact that diets high in fat often tend to be low in fiber, unbalanced in nutrients, and excessive in calories.

It is not the high fat but rather the low fiber, excessive calories, and deficient nutrient intake that presents a risk. Such deficiencies arise from diets lacking enough vegetables. Dietary fiber, especially the soluble kind, is important for the proper maintenance of blood sugar. It also helps to maintain a healthy balance of bacteria in the intestines and to lower the bad type of cholesterol, LDL (low-density lipoprotein). So once again, don't be so concerned about eating too much fat. Instead, make sure that your diet contains an abundance of fiber in the form of vegetables.

PROTEIN

Protein, along with fat, is what your body is made of. It forms most of your body's structural material and is also critically involved in most of the biochemical processes going on around the clock in your physiology. Your cells need your diet to contain enough high-quality protein in order to make muscle tissue and bone, repair damaged organs, maintain sugar stores (glycogen), and produce hormones, enzymes, immunoglobulins, and brain neurotransmitters.

Unfortunately, due to the popularity of vegetarian eating, many health-conscious people have been led to believe that meats, eggs, and dairy are unhealthy for them. Additionally, since Nature designed meat and fat to travel together, the low-fat frenzy has also resulted in a decrease in protein intake.

As I mentioned before, there are eight *essential* amino acids (components of proteins) that must be in optimal amounts in the diet in order to sustain life. An insufficient intake of high-quality dietary protein results in chronic infections, low blood sugar, hormonal deficiencies, attention deficit syndrome, osteoporosis, arthritis, immune deficiencies, and virtually every other degenerative disease associated with aging.

The preferred protein sources for those with diabetes are eggs, dairy, and meats. These are the only protein sources that are referred to as "complete proteins," meaning that they contain all eight essential amino acids. Vegetarian sources of protein are not complete. Since no single source of protein is totally adequate, make sure you eat a variety of these foods.

Also, make sure that you eat a significant amount of protein with virtually every meal. And keep in mind that the more you exercise or exert yourself, the more protein you will need.

The recommended dietary allowance (RDA) for protein for an average-size person is 50 grams per day, but this is a lot less than what appears to be the minimum amount for optimal function. Studies have shown that a total protein intake equaling about 0.7 grams per pound of body weight facilitates weight loss and fat reduction in obese persons. This amounts to 100 grams for a 160-pound person and 150 grams for a person weighing 240 pounds. Other studies have shown that the ideal protein intake required for exercise-induced muscle growth is more in the order of 200 grams per day.

Besides providing eight essential substrates that your body needs to live on, protein has some other very important effects, particularly for the treatment and prevention of diabetes. For example, one of the most important amino acids for diabetics is carnitine. Carnitine not only helps to prevent diabetes, but also lowers elevated triglycerides and cholesterol in diabetics, and can be used therapeutically to alleviate the pain associated with diabetic neuropathy. I will present even more information on the properties of carnitine in Chapter 7.

The amino acid compounds alpha-ketoglutarate and N-acetylcysteine are also especially important for diabetics. Alpha-ketoglutarate enhances the therapeutic effectiveness of insulin and other diabetic medications by improving insulin sensitivity, and N-acetylcysteine helps to prevent diabetic neuropathy.

Protein intake also affects hormone function by influencing whether a hormone is "bound" or not. Unbound hormones are those not molecularly bound to certain proteins. The distinction is important, because when a hormone is bound, it is inactivated and can't perform its functions.

Research has shown that a high intake of dietary protein in general has a very important effect on the hormone profile of diabetics by increasing unbound testosterone levels. This effect is probably secondary to the fact that a high intake of proteins has been found to lower sex hormone binding globulin (SHBG) levels. As its name suggests, SHBG is a protein that binds up the sex hormones so that they cannot exert their effects. Conversely, an insufficient intake of proteins increases the SHBG levels.

Additionally, high protein intake stimulates the production of insulin-like growth factor-1(IGF-1). IGF-1, which I will discuss in Chapter 12, is an important hormone for diabetics.

One worry I often hear from my patients concerns high protein intake and osteoporosis. This is because up until about 1997, it was thought that an excessive consumption of proteins increased the risk of osteoporosis by increasing the loss of calcium from the bones. In fact, studies have shown quite the opposite. Dietary protein turns out to enhance the absorption of calcium. For example, a study undertaken in 1997 demonstrated that urinary calcium loss was no higher in people consuming a whopping 450 grams of protein per day than in people consuming a miniscule 5 grams of protein per day.

A further study demonstrated that women with the highest daily consumption of dietary protein (about 90 grams or more) experienced the lowest number of hip fractures, compared to women who consumed 50 grams per day or less. These studies show that if you are really interested in the prevention of osteoporosis, the more protein you have in your diet, the stronger your bones will be.

SOME GENERAL RECOMMENDATIONS

So, to sum it up, here are the basic dietary guidelines that you can rely on to keep you strong, healthy, and free of diabetes:

- Avoid all hydrogenated and partially hydrogenated fats.

- Avoid high-carbohydrate foods such as grains, sugars, fruit, tubers, and legumes, strictly. Remember, there are no essential carbohydrates, and they are poison to your diabetic metabolism. The minimal amounts of carbohydrates found in dairy, meats, and vegetables are inconsequential.

- Eat all the animal protein and "above-ground" vegetables that you want, with the largest portion of your plate covered with vegetables. This will guarantee that you get enough fiber and high-quality protein.

- Eat the preferred sources of protein, which are, in order: omega-3 eggs, fish and shellfish, lamb, grass-fed beef and poultry, and dairy.

- Eat only as much as you need to. Do not eat more calories than your body requires! Since fats are so high in calories, this often also means decreasing calories by decreasing fat intake. Bio-Energy Testing can tell you exactly what your optimum caloric intake is.

- Drink one glass of water before you eat, and at least four glasses at other times during the day.

- As much as possible, avoid manmade processed foods. There is a reason they are called junk food.

- Particularly avoid reduced-fat foods.

- Use PAM cooking spray, lecithin, olive oil, or butter for oils when you cook.

- Avoid deep-fried foods. Learn to lightly sauté foods in olive oil or butter.

- Never use margarine, shortening, hydrogenated or partially hydrogenated oils, or the "foods" that contain them.

- Keep your breakfasts and lunches light, and make supper the biggest meal of the day. Except in persons who have very physical jobs, I recommend as a routine not eating breakfast at all. The truth is that as long as diabetics insure that their liver function is optimal, they do great on fasts. Those taking insulin would need to adjust their doses accordingly.

- Chew your food well. The food should be close to liquid when you swallow it.

- Eat slowly. And enjoy what you eat.

• Avoid going to sleep for at least three hours after supper. This means eating supper early, say around 6:00 P.M. Three hours is enough time for your body to digest the meal. If you are tired before that time, lie down and rest. But try not to fall asleep. You cannot fully digest your food while you sleep, and this will ultimately lead to increased toxicity and weight gain.

WHAT'S THE BEST WEIGHT-LOSS DIET?

Let me end this chapter by discussing a very interesting article that appeared in the January 5, 2005, edition of the *Journal of the American Medical Association.* Although the article, entitled "Comparison of the Atkins, Ornish, Weight Watchers, and Zone Diets for Weight Loss and Heart Disease Risk Reduction," specifically dealt with weight loss, the findings have great significance to our subject of diabetes. It is important, first, because in large part diabetes is caused by obesity, and also because in order to lose weight patients have to cause their bodies to shift back from glucose metabolism to fat metabolism.

As soon as I saw this article on the journal cover, I just knew that I was finally going to get the inside scoop on the low-fat-versus-low-carbohydrate controversy. And so with baited breath I enthusiastically began reading.

The article first pointed out that there are more than 1,000 books currently available on weight loss, covering everything from eating grapefruits for the rest of your life to living on air instead of food. The public's interest has been further fueled by an almost daily barrage of cover stories from major news magazines, television debates, and cautionary statements regarding the effectiveness and safety of various diets. The authors (Michael L. Dansinger, Joi Augustin Gleason, John L. Griffith, et al.) state that there have been very few studies aimed at looking at the relative merits of the most popular of the weight-loss diets. They, therefore, leaped into this gap and conducted a one-year study comparing the "realistic clinical effectiveness and sustainability for weight loss and cardiac risk reduction" for the four most popular diets.

They enlisted 160 individuals, all of whom were overweight and had high blood pressure, elevated blood lipids, or elevated blood sugar. Then, they divided the participants into four groups of 40 people, and assigned each group to a popular diet. The Atkins group had no calorie restriction, but was limited to 20 grams of carbohydrate per day, which gradually increased to 50 grams per day. The Weight Watchers group was aimed strictly at limiting calories, regardless of ther source. The Ornish group was the low-fat group. They were assigned to a vegetarian diet that contained only 10 percent of calories from fat. Finally, the Zone group was given a "balanced diet" that involved eliminating simple carbohydrates such as flour and sugar, a 20 percent reduction in total carbohydrate calories, and a more or less normal intake of both fat and protein.

Each group met for instruction and support every two weeks for the first two months, and was instructed to take a multivitamin and to exercise at least sixty minutes per week. Now here's where it starts to get interesting.

Each group was asked to follow their diet plan strictly for only the first two months. After that, they were asked to follow the diet "according to their own self-determined interest level." In other words, after the first two months they could cheat as much as they wanted to. The idea was to evaluate not only if one diet was more effective at creating positive medical changes, but also to see if any particular diet was more effective at maintaining compliance. So let's see what happened.

AND THE WINNER IS . . .

First of all, let's take a look at how well these study subjects stuck to their programs. It was remarkable how equally poor all four groups were at following the diet protocols they were assigned to. The Atkins and Zone groups reported following their respective diets only about 70 percent of the time during the first month. The Weight Watchers and Ornish groups were even poorer. They only followed their respective plans 60 percent of the time. The second month was worse yet, with all four groups complying about 10 percent less than they did the first month. Then after the first two months it all went to heck in a hand basket, so that by the sixth month subjects were only following their programs about 30 percent of the time.

In summary, all diets were practically identical in terms of subjects' willingness to adhere to them. It was pointed out that in each group there was a minority of individuals who were exceptionally good at maintaining the discipline necessary for success, and for these individuals the results were much better than for the rest. The authors concluded that in order "to optimally manage a national epidemic of excess body weight and associated risk factors, practical techniques to increase dietary adherence are urgently needed." In other words, there seems to be a great lack of motivation and/or discipline when it comes to altering our cherished eating habits.

So since no one really followed any of the diets much after the first two months, let's take a look at how successful the four diets were at the end of the initial two months. First of all, in terms of weight loss, the winner was . . . no one. All diets were equally effective at producing the same level of weight loss.

How about blood lipids? The clear winner here was the Zone diet, with the Atkins diet running a tight second. The Weight Watchers group and the Ornish low-fat group ran way behind in this department. In terms of blood pressure, Atkins, Zone, and Weight Watchers were all tied, with Ornish relatively ineffective at lowering blood pressure.

As we have seen, insulin and blood sugar levels are the major factors contributing to diabetes. Both of the low-carbohydrate groups, the Atkins and the Zone groups, outperformed the other groups by 3:1 in lowering insulin levels, and by 2:1 in lowering blood sugar. So much for the vegetarian, low-fat concept.

Overall then, at the two-month interval, although all groups were equally effective at lowering weight, only the Atkins and Zone groups stood out in regard to lowering diabetes risk. So what's it all about, Alfie? What conclusions can reasonably be drawn from this very interesting study? Three things occur to me.

One, no matter what positive changes a person needs to make to his diet, it is imperative that he thoroughly commit to his program for a minimum of six months. I have found that it takes about six months for most people to completely adapt to a new way of eating. Anything less is unlikely to be more than a simple waste of time. During that six-month period, I have also found that it is often necessary to meet with the patient at least every three to four weeks to offer encouragement and support. Similarly, the patients who do best are uniformly those who receive the most support at home. It's pretty hard to stick to a healthy diet when everyone else in the house is eating something else.

Secondly, of all the various ways to decrease diabetes risk and lose weight at the same time, the most important single factor is decreasing carbohydrate intake. The rather dramatic enhanced effectiveness of both the Atkins and the Zone diets, both of which restrict carbohydrates, underlines this point. The United States government's ridiculous food pyramid, which strongly emphasizes carbohydrates over fats and proteins, coupled with our modern-day acceptance of carbohydrates as a major food source leaves us with a diet that is both unnatural and quite unhealthy.

Lastly, no one of these four diets is universally effective. Rather, they each share a part of the total truth. The overall goal for ultimate long-term sustained success would be to include the good features of each one of these programs. In other words, not only limit carbohydrates á la Zone and Atkins, but also limit fat and total calories á la Ornish and Weight Watchers. Just doing one without paying heed to the others is a recipe for failure.

As a population we have become accustomed to supersizing not only our carbohydrate intake, but our fat and calorie intakes as well. Real success in this country will only happen when all three of these factors are considered.

CHAPTER 7

STEP TWO:
Supplements

What nature delivers to us is never stale.
Because what nature creates has eternity in it.
—ISAAC BASHEVIS SINGER, AUTHOR (1904–1991)

Supplements are critical for both energy production and optimal fat metabolism. As such, they play a vital role not only in preventing diabetes and the complications associated with diabetes, but also in actually improving blood sugar control.

Years ago when I discussed the subject of supplements, I had to go way out of my way to convince patients and physicians alike that they weren't dangerous, not to mention that they were needed. This was because the medical establishment was firmly convinced that all the nutrition anyone needed to be healthy could be found in foods. They were adamant believers that the only effect of supplements was to produce "expensive urine."

Fortunately, the advocates of this ridiculous assumption have now had to back down and accept that the proof is incontrovertible—supplements are not only helpful, they are essential to optimum health. Over the past ten years there have been many published studies to verify this fact, but a relatively recent article in one of the most prestigious medical journals in the country really drove the point home.

I'm referring to an article published in the *Journal of the American Medical Association* (*JAMA*) entitled "Vitamins for Chronic Disease Prevention in Adults."[1] This article stresses several points that are essential for understanding why nutritional supplements are so necessary.

First, the authors, both from Harvard Medical School, note that there is a very distinct difference between taking the minimal amount of a nutrient to prevent a deficiency syndrome and taking the correct amount of a nutrient to bring about optimal health. This idea is not new. One of the greatest scientific minds of the twentieth century, Linus Pauling, coined the term "orthomolecular medicine" forty years ago to refer to this very same concept. "Ortho-" is Greek for "correct," and by "molecular" he was referring to substances naturally found in the body such as vitamins, hormones, and so on.

The name Linus Pauling is virtually synonymous with the concept of using doses of vitamin C, in order to optimize health, thousands of times in excess of the doses required to prevent scurvy, a vitamin C deficiency disease. Nobody who ever knew Dr. Pauling was surprised when his ortho-molecular theories were validated forty years later, because everyone knows that it is typical for geniuses to be years ahead of their time.

The authors of the *JAMA* article go on to explain why Pauling was right by noting that larger-than-normal doses of nutrients than those obtained through diet alone are necessary to prevent the chronic diseases of aging. To quote the professors on this point, "Most people do not con-sume an optimal amount of all vitamins by diet alone." Their advice: "It appears prudent for all adults to take vitamin supplements." Based on what I have known and seen during more than thirty years of medicine, I would take it a step further and state that it is imprudent and risky not to take supplementary vitamins and minerals.

Of course, one of the diseases that is very much affected by nutrient supplementation is diabetes. So now that it has been officially acknowl-edged that supplements maximize health, let's take a look at which supplements are especially useful for the prevention and treatment of diabetes.

There are seven basic problem areas associated with diabetes in which supplements can be effective. Of course, two of these areas have to do with what I believe are the basic causes of diabetes, namely decreased energy production and decreased fat metabolism. The right supplements can be very effective in correcting both of these disorders. Supplements can also be used to increase or improve insulin sensitivity, liver function, insulin output, adrenal function, and sleep.

Let's start with energy production.

SUPPLEMENTS TO AID OXYGEN METABOLISM

As you have seen, all energy production, and hence the very center of life itself, comes from oxygen metabolism—the conversion of oxygen to water. But this process doesn't just happen in a vacuum. It is a very delicate process that touches on the very mystery of life itself, and which involves a great many nutritional cofactors, that is, special nutrients that are critically necessary in order for the body to use oxygen. As energy needs increase because of everyday life stress, detoxification from ever-increasing environmental exposure to toxic materials, allergens, illness, and so on, these nutritional cofactors get used up at such a rapid rate that they often become deficient. To make matters even worse, several studies have shown that due to a combination of decreased nutrient contents of foods and poor eating habits, most Americans cannot meet their nutritional needs by diet alone. Thus, nutritional supplements, which were once considered by those in the medical community to be unnecessary, are now deemed to be a requirement for optimal health and energy production.

Iron

Perhaps the first nutrient that comes to mind when considering oxygen metabolism is iron. Iron plays two major roles. One, it is the central element in hemoglobin, which is the molecule that carries oxygen in the blood down to the levels of the cells. In cases of iron deficiency, hemoglobin becomes unable to deliver oxygen, and oxygen metabolism decreases as a result.

The other important role of iron is in the mitochondria of the cells. There is a critical enzyme that must be present for oxygen to be metabolized and, thereby, produce energy in what is called the electron transfer system. This enzyme is called cytochrome oxidase, and its activity is completely dependent on iron being present.

Iron deficiency is actually much more common than one would think. Women are especially prone to iron deficiency because they lose iron during their menses. Furthermore, due to a fairly common inherited condition called celiac sprue, many people are unable to adequately absorb iron from their foods.

Unfortunately, some physicians equate iron deficiency with iron deficiency anemia to the point that they believe that iron deficiency does not exist in the absence of anemia. Thus, even if the patient's iron levels are subnormal, they will refrain from prescribing iron unless an actual anemia, meaning an abnormal decrease in red blood cells, is present. The rationale is that although iron is so centrally important to oxygen metabolism, it is also such a potent propagator of free-radical damage that too much iron is a situation they want to be sure to avoid. Hence, I believe many people who are iron deficient end up without treatment.

There are two good ways to avoid this problem. One is simply to undergo Bio-Energy Testing. If there is an iron deficiency, the patient will demonstrate a decrease in energy production. This is the best way to screen for iron deficiency. If iron deficiency is suspected, then some follow-up tests can be used to clarify the situation. The first test would look for the presence of an iron-deficiency anemia. This is easily done by performing a CBC (complete blood count). If there is no anemia present, then testing blood iron levels is the next step. Obviously, if blood iron levels are low, then there is a likelihood of iron deficiency even if there is no anemia.

The second way to avoid undiagnosed iron deficiency is to get a blood test that measures levels of serum ferritin. In cases of iron deficiency, the serum ferritin is often quite low. If you suspect that your iron levels may be low either through Bio-Energy Testing or because you are tired or fatigued, and your serum ferritin is below 30, a trial of iron supplementation is warranted.

Administer iron supplements for two months and have your ferritin levels rechecked. If they have not gone above 80, the odds are that you had iron deficiency. I routinely check the ferritin levels of all of my patients, whether they have diabetes or not, because fairly often I find a patient with either too much or too little iron, and both of these conditions will decrease oxygen metabolism.

Ideally, ferritin levels should be between 30 and 100 nanograms per milliliter (ng/ml), so lower than 30 ng/ml indicates iron deficiency. As part of a general preventive strategy, I recommend that my female patients who are still menstruating take 30 milligrams (mg) of iron per day during their period. I do not recommend that men take iron unless an iron deficiency has been demonstrated.

Aiding Oxygen Delivery

After oxygen is taken up by hemoglobin, it is carried through the circulation until it finally arrives at its destination, the cells. At that point an enzyme by the name of 2,3 DPG displaces the oxygen molecule from hemoglobin and thereby allows it to diffuse into the surrounding cells. Diabetics are routinely deficient in 2,3 DPG, and this deficiency prevents a substantial amount of oxygen from being released into the cells. The delivery truck has arrived, but it is not dropping off the oxygen, which is basically the same as if the truck had not arrived in the first place. Deficiency in 2,3 DPG, therefore, significantly impairs oxygen consumption and energy production in diabetics.

The enzyme 2,3 DPG is formed in red blood cells through the action of niacin (vitamin B_3) and the amino acid molecule glutathione. Both niacin and glutathione can easily become depleted, and often need to be supplemented.

Niacin

One of the more common signs of niacin deficiency is an elevated serum triglyceride level, which is often seen in diabetics. To help with 2,3 DPG synthesis, I routinely give all my patients a minimum of 100 mg niacin per day, and prescribe much more than this for many of them. Exercise has also been found to appreciably increase the formation of 2,3 DPG.

N-Acetylcysteine

Replenishing glutathione is a slightly different matter than just taking glutathione capsules, because glutathione is only very poorly absorbed from the gastrointestinal tract. In fact, the only really effective way to increase glutathione levels is to take the amino acid N-acetylcysteine, which is efficiently absorbed and will quickly be converted into glutathione by the liver. I routinely give my patients 50–100 mg of N-acetylcysteine per day.

Aiding Oxygen Metabolism in the Cells

After the oxygen is released from hemoglobin because of the action of 2,3 DPG, it then diffuses into the cell and is taken into the mitochondria. In the mitochondria it will be combined with hydrogen to form water and energy. The hydrogen molecule will be supplied by the citric acid cycle, also called the Krebs cycle after its discoverer H. A. Krebs. In this biochemical cycle, the hydrocarbon molecules that make up the fat and carbohydrate in our diets are broken down into carbon dioxide and hydrogen, and it is this hydrogen atom that is subsequently combined with oxygen. Thus, oxygen can be converted to energy only as long as the Krebs cycle is able to supply hydrogen, and this is why the function of the Krebs cycle is absolutely essential to life.

Many nutrients are involved in the Krebs cycle, but the ones that are most notable are folic acid, niacin, magnesium, manganese, iron, malic acid, lipoic acid, thiamine (vitamin B_1), and alpha-ketoglutaric acid. These nutrients are used up rapidly due to their energy-supplying role, and often need to be replaced. Niacin and iron have already been discussed.

Magnesium

Magnesium's role in energy production stems from its participation as an essential cofactor not only in the Krebs cycle, but also for almost all of the enzymes involved in the production of energy. People who start magnesium supplementation often notice a significant improvement in their energy levels within four to ten days. I routinely prescribe 600 mg of magnesium per day to my patients, and I often find I need even more than this to replenish depleted reserves.

Manganese

Manganese not only serves an essential role in the Krebs cycle, but due to its ability to activate the enzymes involved in the process of sugar metabolism, it is particularly valuable in diabetes. In fact, because diabetics have such great demand for manganese, it is not surprising that a study published in the *American Journal of Clinical Nutrition* in 1987 found that diabetics are generally found to have approximately half the levels of manganese of nondiabetics.[2] I routinely give my patients 10 mg of manganese per day to insure that they are getting enough.

Malic Acid and Alpha-Ketoglutaric Acid

Malic acid and alpha-ketoglutaric acid are key amino acids that are particularly important in the Krebs cycle. Supplemental malic acid is often critical for maximum energy production, and studies have shown that doses between 3 and 6 grams are able to increase energy production, even in athletes. In those with diabetes, its effect tends to be even more dramatic, and it often alleviates fatigue and increases stamina.

Like malic acid, alpha-ketoglutaric acid improves athletic performance through its effect on the Krebs cycle, but it also enhances the therapeutic effectiveness of insulin in both type 1 and type 2 diabetes. Effective doses for alpha-ketoglutarate range from 1,800–2,200 mg per day. I regularly find that both of these nutrients are needed to adequately optimize energy levels in my diabetic patients.

Lipoic Acid and Thiamine

Lipoic acid and thiamine (vitamin B_1) serve central roles in the Krebs cycle by being the nutrients essential for the production of acetyl-coenzyme A, the substance that starts the cycle. Without adequate levels of acetyl-coenzyme A, the Krebs cycle cannot even get off the ground. In a 1996 article that appeared in the diabetic journal *Diabetologia*, the authors found that thiamine was absolutely critical for the optimum function of the Krebs cycle.[3] Thiamine is so critical that in the event that it is depleted, the body will form dangerous levels of lactic acid from the very same molecule that thiamine converts into acetyl-coenzyme A. I routinely give my patients 100 mg of thiamine per day.

Lipoic acid is important to anybody over the age of fifty, and this is especially true of those with diabetes. Research has shown that lipoic acid helps to prevent the onset of diabetes; it improves blood sugar control; it reduces the incidence of cataracts in diabetics; it prevents the damage to the kidneys, which is a common diabetes complication; and it has been shown to prevent the peripheral neuropathy that is so common in those with diabetes. In fact, I have used lipoic acid with fairly good success to treat diabetic neuropathy in doses of up to 200 mg three times per day. In the absence of neuropathy, however, I typically use doses of around 300 to 400 mg per day.

Helping Convert Oxygen to Energy

Once the Krebs cycle has made a hydrogen atom available, then the actual process that combines oxygen with hydrogen to form water and energy can begin. This happens in the mitochondria's electron transfer system, and the very first enzyme involved in this system is known as coenzyme Q_{10}, or CoQ_{10} for short.

Approximately 50 percent of the body's total CoQ_{10} content is found in the mitochondria. So important is CoQ_{10} to energy production that in its absence, energy production completely shuts down, and death quickly ensues.

Even more impressive is that supplements of CoQ_{10} can be used to enhance mitochondrial function even when a deficiency is not present.

Note, for example, a study published in *Cellular Molecular Biology* of six patients who were given 150 mg of CoQ_{10} per day for six months. Although these patients all had mitochondrial disorders, they were not found to be deficient in CoQ_{10}. Nonetheless, the authors found that "increased coenzyme Q_{10} concentration in the mitochondrial membrane increases the efficiency of oxidative phosphorylation [that is, the electron transfer system] independently of enzyme deficit."[4] What all that means is that CoQ_{10} is so important to cellular function that even when a deficiency is not present, supplementary CoQ_{10} is still able to improve energy production.

Other studies have shown that CoQ_{10} has been found to reverse the accelerated death of cells known as apoptosis, which is a primary cause of the aging process. CoQ_{10} is also especially important for diabetics. Articles appearing in the *Journal of Medicine*,[5] and in the *Journal of Vitaminology*[6] have demonstrated the following:

- Eight percent of diabetes patients are deficient in CoQ_{10}.

- CoQ_{10} reduces blood sugar levels by at least 30 percent in nondiabetic patients, and reduces it by at least 20 percent in more than a third of all diabetics.

- Many of the complications associated with diabetes worsen when a deficiency of CoQ_{10} is present.

Other studies have shown that CoQ_{10} at only 120 mg per day is also very effective in decreasing the insulin resistance that causes diabetes in the first place.

CoQ_{10} and all of the other components of the electron transfer system are attached to and work from a membrane in the mitochondria made of a fat called cardiolipin. I make a point of this because the presence of cardiolipin is essential for the functioning of all the elements of the electron transfer system, and studies have shown that it becomes damaged and destroyed as we get older due to the action of free-radical molecules. Free-radical molecules are found in very high numbers in the mitochondria.

The damage caused by free-radical activity is prevented through the action of antioxidant nutrients such as vitamin C, vitamin E, and glutathione. This protection is extremely important in the mitochondria in order to maintain a youthful level of energy production. This is why taking these antioxidant nutrients is an essential aspect of maintaining maximum energy production, decreasing the rate of aging, and preventing and treating diabetes. In this regard, CoQ_{10} becomes even more important, because in addition to its other functions, it is also the principal antioxidant in the mitochondria. I routinely prescribe for my patients the following daily intake of these critical supplements: 100–200 mg CoQ_{10}, 2,000 mg vitamin C, 400 IU (international units) vitamin E, and 100 mg N-acetylcysteine (to raise glutathione levels).

In the event that cardiolipin is already damaged, several animal studies have indicated that the levels of this fat can be restored by combining lipoic acid with the amino acid L-carnitine. In fact, in a very interesting article with the ambitious title "The Effect of Aging and Acetyl-L-Carnitine on the Activity of the Phosphate Carrier and on the Phospholipid Composition [cardiolipin] in Rat Heart Mitochondria," the authors note that the mitochondrial level of cardiolipin steadily decreases with aging. More important, however, they found that "treatment of aged rats with acetyl-L-carnitine restored the level of cardiolipin to that of young rats."[7] I will tell you more about carnitine in just a moment, but suffice it to say that I find L-carnitine to be an extremely useful supplement, partly because it acts to restore damaged cardiolipin. I routinely give my diabetic and prediabetic patients anywhere from 1,000 to 3,000 mg of acetyl-L-carnitine each day.

SUPPLEMENTS TO INCREASE FAT METABOLISM

The second major way supplements can help to prevent, treat, and even reverse diabetes is by increasing fat metabolism. Carnitine also plays a major role in this respect, as do niacin and lipoic acid, two nutrients that work together to increase fat metabolism. This duo is critical to the operation of the process referred to as beta-oxidation, wherein fat molecules are broken down in the cell until they are small enough to be escorted by carnitine into the mitochondria. Finally, there are several herbal supplements that are useful aids to fat metabolism.

L-Carnitine

L-carnitine plays a key role in fat metabolism because without it, it would be impossible to transport fat into the mitochondria to be converted into energy. To perform this critical function, carnitine combines with a molecule of fat and a molecule of acetyl-coenzyme A to make a complex that can penetrate the membrane of the mitochondria. Inside the mitochondria, the complex liberates the carnitine, which then moves back to the outside of the membrane so it is able to repeat the process. Carnitine, thus, serves as a continuous shuttle to carry fat molecules into the mitochondria. Without enough carnitine present, the cells would not be able to metabolize fat at all because it would not be able to get past the membrane. Effective doses of carnitine are from 1,000 mg to 3,000 mg per day.

Niacin

I am completely convinced, after successfully using therapeutic doses of niacin for the past twenty years in thousands of patients with various clinical disorders, that niacin is a nutrient that the majority of the population is very much in need of. Niacin is so critical to fat metabolism that deficiencies of it are the single most common cause of elevated blood fats such as triglycerides and cholesterol.

One thing that you must be aware of if you take sufficient quantities of niacin is that it causes a "flushing" or burning sensation during the first several weeks of use. This sensation begins about twenty minutes after it is ingested and usually lasts about twenty to twenty-five minutes. During this time, patients will feel a flushed, burning, pins-and-needles type of reaction in the face and sometimes all over the body. Occasionally, the sensation is quite uncomfortable, but it is important to realize that it is not dangerous and does not represent any kind of allergic reaction. I simply consider it to be a detoxification reaction, because after the first few weeks of taking niacin, the symptoms decrease to a very tolerable level or will disappear entirely. I like giving niacin in a routine dose of 100 mg per day, but when there are indications for additional need such as increased triglyceride and/or decreased HDL cholesterol levels, I often use up to 1,500 mg per day.

Lipoic Acid

Lipoic acid, like niacin, is another one of those nutrients on my all-time top one hundred list because it is a cofactor in so many different reactions. It is a major antioxidant, working with vitamins C and E and CoQ_{10} to protect both cardiolipin and mitochondrial DNA from free-radical damage. It also acts as a heavy metal chelator, removing such toxic metals as lead, arsenic, cadmium, and mercury from the body.

Lipoic acid also plays a major role in energy production. This last attribute is exemplified in a 1995 study published in the *Journal of Neurology*. In this study, a patient was treated with 600 mg of lipoic acid daily for only one month. The net result was a full 72 percent increase in energy production! Seven months later even greater improvement was noted. The researchers concluded, "Our results indicate that treatment with lipoic acid caused a relevant increase in levels of energy available in brain and skeletal muscle during exercise."[8]

Lipoic acid is particularly valuable in both the prevention and treatment of diabetes. It has been shown to improve the transport and the utilization of glucose in various experimental and animal models, which is just a long-winded way of saying that it increases insulin sensitivity. This was really brought home in a 1999 study. In this study, seventy-four patients with type 2 diabetes were treated with either a placebo capsule or lipoic acid. After only four weeks, the effects on insulin sensitivity of lipoic acid versus placebo treatment were compared. The authors say it plainly, "The results suggest that oral administration of alpha-lipoic acid can improve insulin sensitivity in patients with type 2 diabetes."[9]

The literature also shows that lipoic acid prevents and alleviates many of the detrimental complications caused by both type 1 and type 2 diabetes. For example, it

- Helps to prevent the onset of type 1 diabetes;

- Reduces the incidence of cataracts, a common problem in diabetes;

- Prevents the damage to the kidneys (diabetic nephropathy), another complication of diabetes;

- Prevents the burning pain in the feet that is a common side effect of diabetes called neuropathy.

In my opinion, supplementary lipoic acid should be considered an absolutely essential part of any comprehensive treatment and prevention strategy for diabetes. I routinely prescribe 300 to 600 mg lipoic acid per day.

Herbal Supplements

In addition to the above nutrients, there are also a number of herbal products that can dramatically increase fat metabolism. I routinely recommend the following combination one to two times per day, not only for my diabetic patients but for any of my patients whose ability to burn fat is less than optimal:

- *Camellia sinensis* extract: 250–500 mg

- *Citrus aurantium* extract: 250–500 mg

- *Coleus forskohli* extract (leaf): 50–100 mg

- *Eleutherococcus senticosus* extract (root): 50–100 mg

- *Panax ginseng* extract (root): 50–100 mg

These herbal extracts are even more effective when they are used in combination with the amino acid L-tyrosine. Research has shown that L-tyrosine increases energy production by facilitating the production of the fat-burning hormones thyroxine and norepinephrine. I usually give my patients from 250 to 500 mg of L-tyrosine per day.

SUPPLEMENTS TO INCREASE INSULIN SENSITIVITY

As I'm sure you know by now, increasing insulin sensitivity is a central goal in the prevention and treatment of diabetes. In the last section I discussed how important lipoic acid was in this regard, but there are a number of other supplements that are also very effective, including fish oil, chromium, and vanadium.

Fish Oil

Fish oil is high in omega-3 fat. You might recall that I discussed omega-3 fat along with omega-6 fat in Chapter 6. One of the most important things to remember about these fats is that they play a critical role in the production of hormones called prostaglandins. Different prostaglandins produce opposing effects in the body, so it is very important to maintain a balance of these hormones. Nutritional research has shown that due to the dramatic shift in both our diets and animal-feeding practices over the last hundred years, the balance of fats in our bodies contains about twenty times more omega-6 than it should. Among the many complications of this imbalance is decreased insulin sensitivity.

A very practical way to insure an adequate balance and improve insulin sensitivity is to take an omega-3 supplement such as concentrated fish oil. I routinely prescribe from 1,000 to 3,000 mg of omega-3 fat per day in this form. One thing to note here is that the prostaglandins that are formed from omega-3 fat are ones that are needed to keep the blood thin and freely flowing. This is especially good in terms of preventing heart attacks and strokes, but is not desirable if you are going into surgery. So I always tell my patients to stop eating fish and taking fish oil supplements for at least a week before surgery.

Chromium

Another nutrient that is extremely effective at increasing insulin sensitivity is chromium. R. A. Anderson and colleagues found in their research that 1,000 micrograms (mcg) of chromium per day resulted in a "spectacular" increase in insulin sensitivity in the patients with type 2 diabetes they studied.[10]

Chromium probably has this effect as a result of being the critical element in a compound called glucose tolerance factor (GTF). GTF is composed of one chromium molecule plus two molecules of niacin and one molecule each of the amino acids cysteine, glutamic acid, and glycine.

GTF works in tandem with insulin to regulate blood sugar levels, and also has a primary control effect on cholesterol synthesis and metabolism. GTF has been found to lower total cholesterol levels by 25 percent, increase HDL cholesterol (the "good" one) by up to 18 percent, and decrease LDL cholesterol (the "bad" one) by up to 18 percent. Because of its effect on insulin sensitivity, chromium also lowers elevated triglycerides levels.

For several years, I analyzed both the blood and the cellular chromium levels of all of my patients, and in that time I almost never found a patient with optimal chromium levels. Perhaps this is why I see a huge clinical advantage to chromium supplementation. I routinely prescribe my patients anywhere from 1,000 to 3,000 mcg of chromium per day.

Vanadium

Like chromium, vanadium is another trace mineral that plays an enormous role in the activity of insulin. Vanadium, in the form of vanadyl sulfate, not only improves insulin resistance, but it also has its own insulin effect, which makes it especially useful in diabetics who have low insulin levels.

In one 1996 study published in *Metabolism*, the authors gave eight patients with type 2 diabetes 50 mg of vanadyl sulfate twice a day for four weeks and noted that the "vanadyl sulfate treatment resulted in a 20 percent reduction in average fasting blood sugar."[11] The literature is replete with articles showing similar results. I usually use vanadyl sulfate in my patients with diabetes only when their blood sugar control is not perfect and their insulin levels are lower than 10 microunits per milliliter (mU/ml). When this happens, I call the condition low-insulin diabetes, and I will routinely prescribe 50 mg to be taken two to three times per day.

Herbal Supplements

There are several herbs that can be very helpful in improving insulin sensitivity. One of them, *Galega officinalis*, contains an ingredient called guanidine from which the diabetic drug metformin is produced. I use an extract of the leaf that is standardized to 20 percent guanylhydrazine. Another valuable herb is *Mormodica charantia*, also known as bitter melon. Both of these herbs increase insulin sensitivity and, as a result, improve glucose tolerance in diabetes.

For my patients, I routinely prescribe 320 mg of a 4:1 extract of *Mormodica charantia*, along with 80 mg of *Galega officinalis* extract twice a day. At these doses, I have found that, used by themselves, these herbs offer a modest effect on insulin sensitivity, but when combined with other supplements in this chapter, particularly chromium, lipoic acid, vanadium, fish oil, and carnitine, they can really make a difference.

SUPPLEMENTS TO INCREASE LIVER FUNCTION

As you will learn in Chapter 9, optimal liver function is crucial for the prevention and treatment of diabetes. The liver is constantly synthesizing vital compounds, metabolizing and regulating hormone levels, maintaining blood sugar control, and detoxifying the entire body. In order to accomplish all these tasks, it uses up a tremendous amount of nutrients, especially the B vitamins and the antioxidants. It also requires substantial levels of magnesium, zinc, selenium, manganese, potassium, and copper.

Look at the list of nutrients and their doses in the QuickStart-DM formula, detailed in Appendix A of this book, and you will have a complete list of all the supplements, along with doses, needed to provide ultimate support for the liver.

SUPPLEMENTS TO INCREASE INSULIN OUTPUT

As far as I know, there is only one nutritional supplement that actually has the capability of increasing the pancreatic output of insulin—*Gymnema sylvestre*. It is an extract of the leaves of the plant that contains a substance known as GS4 that is responsible for its action.

In a 1990 study, the effectiveness of GS4 in controlling blood sugar was investigated in twenty-two patients with type 2 diabetes who were already on conventional oral medications. A dosage of 400 mg per day of GS4 was administered for eighteen to twenty months as a supplement to their medications. During GS4 supplementation, the researchers noted a significant reduction in blood sugar and hemoglobin A1c, and the medications were able to be decreased in every patient. Five of the patients were able to discontinue their medications altogether and maintain blood sugar control with GS4 alone.[12]

The reason that GS4 appears to work so well is twofold. First, as other studies using animal models have shown, over time, often twelve to eighteen months, GS4 actually brings about an increase in the number of islet cells in the pancreas. GS4, it turns out, has a regeneration and repair effect on the islet cells, which had been previously destroyed by free-radical activity.

Second, given that insulin levels have been shown to increase after administration of GS4, it seems to have a direct stimulatory effect on the pancreas, causing it to produce more insulin. Of course, any increase in insulin output from an already "tired" pancreas may lead to islet-cell destruction from free radicals, so it is especially important when taking *Gymnema sylvestre* to make sure to take plenty of antioxidant nutrients.

I routinely prescribe my low-insulin-diabetes patients, that is, those with insulin levels under 10 mU/ml, anywhere from 600 to 1,200 mg per day of *Gymnema sylvestre* extract standardized to contain 24 percent gymnemic acids. This supplies about 150 to 300 mg of gymnemic acids per day.

SUPPLEMENTS TO INCREASE ADRENAL FUNCTION

The adrenal hormone cortisol is vital for the prevention of diabetes. This miracle hormone converts protein to blood sugar thereby maintaining steady blood sugar levels, and is especially important when utilizing all the advantages of a low-carbohydrate diet. Additionally, cortisol, along with the other adrenal hormones, acts to improve total energy production, and in particular acts to improve energy production from fat. Thus, the adrenal hormones all by themselves have the ability to prevent the shift from fat metabolism to glucose metabolism that is at the very heart of what causes diabetes in the first place. So no wonder why I am so adamant about diagnosing adrenal insufficiency in my patients, and aggressively treating it when I find it. Here I present the supplements I have found to be the most helpful in improving adrenal function.

Pantothenic Acid

Pantothenic acid (vitamin B_5), since it is an essential cofactor for the production of most steroid hormones, enhances the body's production of the adrenal hormones cortisol and cortisone. Pantothenic acid is particularly valuable when patients are under stress, whether it be emotional or physical such as pain or illness. I routinely recommend between 500 mg and 2,000 mg of pantothenic acid per day.

DHEA

DHEA (dehydroepiandrosterone) supplementation is another important treatment. DHEA is a steroid hormone produced in the adrenal gland that declines rather significantly as we become older. I discuss DHEA in much greater detail a little later in Chapter 12.

Although it is a hormone, it is sold over the counter. DHEA is essential to the functioning of the immune system and almost every other system studied, but studies have found it to be particularly helpful in cases of adrenal insufficiency. DHEA has been shown to improve mood, exhaustion, and other symptoms common to the disorder. As an extra attraction, research has also demonstrated that supplemental DHEA acts to increase insulin sensitivity in patients with deficient levels.

A word of caution should be added here. DHEA can be converted by the body into the hormones testosterone and estrogen, and as such should probably not be taken by anyone with a history of either breast or prostate cancer, unless the levels of these hormones are being monitored. For the same reason, it can also cause acne and hair loss as well as breast and prostate swelling. In fact, although it is extremely safe when properly used, it is my belief that no one should take DHEA without the direct supervision of a physician who is familiar with it.

Good starting doses for DHEA are in the order of 10 mg per day for women and 25 mg per day for men. Depending on clinical conditions and how the testosterone and estrogen levels are affected, I will often recommend much more than this for my patients.

Licorice

One of my all-time favorite treatments for adrenal insufficiency is *Gly-*

cyrrhiza glabra, more commonly known as licorice. I love licorice. I'm talking about licorice the herb here, not licorice the candy. There is a big difference!

Glycyrrhiza glabra is extremely effective at supporting exhausted adrenal glands because it works in several ways. First of all, it contains natural precursors for the production of adrenal hormones. Second, it possesses activity similar to the adrenal hormone aldosterone, which is often deficient in adrenal insufficiency. And last, it acts to prevent the liver from metabolizing cortisol, and in this way is able to actually increase cortisol levels when they are deficient. I routinely prescribe between 350 mg and 700 mg of *Glycyrrhiza glabra* extract root, standardized for 16 percent glycyrrhizinic acid, once or twice a day.

A word of caution should also be stated here. Although I have found it to be quite uncommon, I have seen a few cases where these doses of licorice have resulted in a modest increase in blood pressure. For this reason, I always have my patients with hypertension monitor their blood pressure while taking licorice. Also, the literature describes potassium loss as a side effect of licorice use, and since those with diabetes are usually already depleted in potassium, I make sure to have diabetic patients supplement with at least 300 mg of potassium per day.

SUPPLEMENTS TO IMPROVE AND INCREASE SLEEP

As you will see in Chapter 10, one of the major contributors to insulin resistance and diabetes is sleep deprivation. Sleep deprivation also results in decreased levels of growth hormone and testosterone, two very important hormones, especially for those with diabetes.

The single most common cause of insomnia and poor-quality sleep is stress and worry. My patients are repeatedly telling me that they have trouble falling asleep, sleep lightly, are easily awakened, and often can't get back to sleep as a result of worrisome thoughts racing through their heads. Often, taking a sedative will help but there are better ways.

To promote good-quality sleep, I routinely recommend that patients take the following about twenty minutes before bedtime:

- Niacinamide: 1,000 mg

- Theanine: 100 mg

- 5-HTP: 100 mg

- Niacin: 10 mg

- Magnesium: 16 mg

- Melatonin: 1.5 mg

Now, let's take a look at the function and effect of each of these supplements.

Niacinamide

The niacinamide form of vitamin B_3 improves the quality of sleep by binding to what are known as the benzodiazepine receptors of the brain. These are the very same receptors that the drug Valium interacts with to cause sedation. When taken before bed, niacinamide is very helpful in causing a mental sedation, allowing you to let go of all those stressful things you have to remember and think over. This results in falling and staying asleep much more easily, and unlike with Valium, no addiction results from taking this B vitamin.

Theanine

I find that a substance found in green tea called theanine is also useful to calm down anxious thoughts and feelings prior to going to sleep. Theanine sedates the brain by increasing the output of relaxing alpha waves, the same wave forms that are predominant during times of extreme relaxation.

5-HTP

5-HTP (5-hydroxytryptophan) is an amino acid that is converted to serotonin in the brain. This conversion is enhanced in the presence of niacin (not niacinamide—they are different), and so taking a little niacin along with 5-HTP improves its effect.

Serotonin is the same brain chemical that is affected by all the new wonder medications for mood and sleep, such as Prozac and Wellbutrin. 5-HTP has the same effects as these medications but without the many side effects, but don't wait for your pharmaceutical representative to tell you. Research has shown that 5-HTP increases total sleep time as well as total REM sleep. A little side benefit here is that by increasing serotonin levels, 5-HTP is also able to decrease cravings for carbohydrates and improve mood stability.

Magnesium

Magnesium is another nutrient that has been studied extensively for its effects on anxiety and insomnia. Animal studies demonstrate that higher brain magnesium content is associated both with improved sleep quality and longer slow-wave sleep episodes. You will learn more about the advantages of slow-wave sleep in Chapter 10. Patient studies show that magnesium, when taken just prior to going to bed, improves the quality of sleep.

Melatonin

Melatonin is a hormone produced in a part of the brain called the pineal gland. Its release into the system is inhibited by light, and so melatonin levels are very low during the day. Then when it becomes dark and we turn out the lights, melatonin is suddenly released and a feeling of sleepiness results. This is one reason why it is so important not to leave any lights on while you are sleeping.

Melatonin is perhaps the single most heavily studied hormone. Supplemental melatonin decreases the proportion of stage 1 sleep (light sleep), while at the same time increasing the proportion of stage 2 sleep, REM sleep. This results in a deeper, more consistent level of sleep with fewer awakenings. It also greatly reduces the amount of movement during sleep, reduces the time it takes to fall asleep, and improves the subjective quality of sleep.

Although melatonin has been found to be safe in doses forty to fifty times the recommended dose, it usually only takes a very small amount of this hormone to improve sleep. Also, occasionally I find that certain people will report sleep disturbances such as excessive dreams and restlessness with melatonin. Others have told me that even at small doses, they find themselves feeling drowsy and oversedated in the morning. In these cases, lowering the dose is usually effective.

Unproven Supplements or Proven Medications?

A few years ago I proposed a bill to the Nevada State Legislature that would have encouraged the use of nutritional supplements by physicians to both treat and prevent disease. I thought it was a good idea because many physicians would like to prescribe nutritional therapies but don't because they are afraid of being criticized by the medical community for practicing "unproven medicine." Judging by the incredible reaction against this bill that came from the state medical association, you would have thought that I was trying to get physicians to put their patients on acid.

I remember one incident in particular: I was discussing the intent of the bill with a physician from the state medical association, who was there to argue against it. He asked me how in the world I dared to use natural substances to treat my patients when there were so few double-blind, controlled studies to verify efficacy. I told him that I did not feel that such studies were always needed, especially in circumstances in which the substances I was using were known to be safe and inexpensive. In such a scenario the worst outcome would be that they just didn't work, in which case I could always use the standard medications anyway.

He said he thought that that was practicing incompetent medicine, and that he would much rather use medications with known dangers and side effects "because at least they are proven, and I know what to expect." I guess I'm grateful that I could never see that kind of logic, because over the years I have been blessed to see so many patients successfully replace their "proven" patent medications and the side effects that went with them with less proven natural supplements.

Supplements are just that. They are supplements. They are not meant to replace medications when medications are really needed, but how in the world are you going to know that a medication is really needed unless you try the supplements first?

A Quick Start Is a Good Start

As you will read later in Chapter 9, I have created a super-supplement duo called QuickStart-DM and Super Fat. Together these two supplements include most of the nutrients that have been discussed in this chapter, providing a convenient, cost-effective way to take these nutrients.

CHAPTER 8

STEP THREE:
Exercise

*"Exercise ferments the humors, casts them into
their proper channels, throws off redundancies,
and helps nature in those secret distributions,
without which the body cannot subsist in its vigor,
nor the soul act with cheerfulness."*

—JOSEPH ADDISON, ESSAYIST, POET, AND POLITICIAN (1672–1719)

Few things perhaps are more misunderstood than exercise. In this country, by focusing primarily on the importance of exercise for young people, we seem to have the whole concept completely backwards. We are almost obsessed with making sure that our kids get plenty of exercise. We make sure they have regular physical education classes—if you've had children in the school system, you know that getting them excused from gym class usually requires something akin to a letter from the Pope. We go to great expense making sure that schools offer a large and diverse sports program, and enthusiastically encourage participation.

The irony in all this is that, while exercise is obviously good for everyone, the primary needs of the under-forty crew are good nutrition and adequate rest. Exercise, per se, is not nearly as critical as it will become later in life. The reason for this is that in this age bracket, the body is still able to maintain its function and repair systems at optimal levels. When you were this age and you sprained your ankle, it only took a few days to recover. Likewise, if you were bedridden for some reason, even for weeks on end, you would lose little to no lean body mass (muscle and bone), because your young body would be able to maintain it.

Somewhere around the age of forty, however, all that starts to change. In your mind you are still the same person, but what you don't recognize is that your physiology is slowing down in some very significant, though subtle, ways. And without really being aware of it, your body's ability to preserve form and function changes. It now *requires* exercise in order to maintain itself.

Because of this principle, as we grow older, unless we regularly exercise, our muscle and bone mass, cardiac output, lung function, and energy production will steadily decrease. As you know by now, decreased energy production is what causes diabetes as well as all of the other diseases and infirmities associated with getting older. Exercise can effectively counter all of these decreases, and in the process, slow down the rate at which you biologically age.

EXERCISE IS NOT OPTIONAL

Go into a health club and who do you see? Not many people over sixty. Mostly you see the younger set, while the majority of the older generation is home actively pursuing some version of couch behavior and thinking to themselves, "I've got to take it easy. I'm too old for that kid stuff."

The truth is just the opposite. They're too old *not* to do that stuff. Exercising is a luxury for the under-forty set, but it is an absolute necessity for the rest of us. Those of us who want to avoid disease, slow down the aging process, and function at a much younger level, need to understand that *regular* exercise is *essential.*

Exercise as a "longevity elixir" has been the focus of an ongoing world-famous study conducted by Stanford researcher Ralph Paffenbarger, Jr., M.D. With updates published over the years in leading medical journals, the study tracks exercise habits and longevity among more than 17,000 Harvard alumni. In a 1986 report for the *New England Journal of Medicine,* Paffenbarger revealed his finding that "for each hour of physical activity, you can expect to live that hour over—and live one or two more hours to boot."[1]

And here's more evidence that demonstrates how vital exercise is, particularly to those over forty years of age:

- According to a study by Ken Cooper, M.D., of the Cooper Institute of Aerobic Research, there are 40 percent fewer heart attacks among women who exercise and 60 percent fewer among exercising males. In another study, Dr. Cooper determined that individuals in the lowest 20 percent bracket of cardiovascular fitness had a death rate three times higher than the fittest group. The study also indicated that men who start exercise, even after the age of sixty, will increase their life expectancy.[2]

- Among postmenopausal women, osteoporosis can be reduced by weight training twice a week. Such exercise increases bone density. It also improves strength and balance, and thereby reduces the risk of falls in the elderly. This lowers the mortality rate because fractured hips from falls are associated with a fairly high death rate.

- A 1994 study in the *Journal of the American Medical Association* points to a decreased incidence of gastrointestinal hemorrhage among elderly people who exercise regularly.[3]

- A recent article in the *Archives of Internal Medicine* demonstrated that men who were physically unfit were almost *three times as likely to die from all causes, including cancer,* even after the researchers accounted for age, smoking, and alcohol use.[4]

- Various studies have shown that exercise reduces the incidence of colon cancer by 50 percent.

- Impotence occurs in 25 percent of all men over the age of sixty-five and is especially common in men with diabetes. Researchers say, however, that men who regularly exercise have a much lower incidence of this problem. If you like sex, you're going to love exercise!

- Exercise is the healthiest way to treat depression. A study reported in the journal *Psychosomatic Medicine* in 2000 concluded not only that exercise provides as much effectiveness against depression as the latest medications, but the long-term results from exercise therapy are actually superior to medication—with no side effects![5]

- Exercise also helps keep Alzheimer's disease, as well as the "usual" mental decline associated with aging, at bay. It is also a very effective treatment for insomnia.

And if all this is true for the average person, it is doubly true for those with prediabetes and diabetes.

DIABETES AND THE BENEFITS OF EXERCISE

There is overwhelming evidence in the scientific literature documenting the incredible efficacy of exercise for diabetes prevention and treatment. For instance, J. G. Lim and colleagues reported their findings in 2004 in the *Singapore Medical Journal:* "Exercise training is an essential component in both the medical management of patients with type 2 diabetes and in preventing the development of diabetes among those at risk. It is particularly important for physicians to recognize patients at risk for diabetes or those who have already developed the pre-diabetic state, as intervention in terms of exercise and other lifestyle changes will reap the greatest benefits at this stage."[6]

Given that exercise has been proven to be essential in the prevention and management of diabetes, it continues to amaze me that virtually none of the diabetics I see are exercising regularly. Most are not even exercising at all! According to Lim et al., the reasons for this dereliction of duty "include patients' lack of knowledge about the benefits of exercise, a lack of motivation, and a lack of clear recommendations from healthcare professionals." I will cover all of these issues in this chapter.

When it comes to improving energy production, there is literally nothing more effective than correct exercise. The truth of the dictum "What you don't use, you lose" becomes increasingly evident the older we get. Unfortunately, the sedentary lifestyle of our modern age, in which we enjoy the best in creature comforts, is killing us. In one study published in 2002 in *Diabetes Care,* the authors demonstrated that men who engaged in three hours per week of moderate exercise were half as likely as their sedentary counterparts to develop prediabetes.[7]

In another study, every two-hour-per-day increment in television watching was associated with a 14 percent increased risk of developing diabetes. On the other hand, each one hour per day spent briskly walking was associated with a 34 percent decrease in diabetes risk.[8]

Keep in mind that none of these studies considered diet as a factor. These remarkable results are solely from exercise. Now let's take a closer look at the some of the benefits of exercise for diabetics, starting with decreased death rate.

Decreased Death Rate

A lack of exercise results in an increased death rate in patients with type 2 diabetes. One recent study revealed an incredible 58 percent reduction in death rate of those with type 2 diabetes who exercised regularly. Exercise has this positive effect because it increases energy production, which leads to decreased blood sugar levels, increased insulin sensitivity, increased muscle strength, decreased blood pressure, improved cholesterol and triglyceride levels, decreased body fat, improved cardiac function, decreased systemic inflammation, and improved arterial elasticity.

Improved Blood Sugar Control and Insulin Sensitivity

Numerous studies show that regular exercise improves blood sugar control. One major factor in this regard is an increased ability of muscle tissue to take up glucose and thus keep the levels lower. Another reason is that exercise induces the synthesis of certain enzymes in the liver that improve the liver's ability to regulate blood sugar. A third reason is that exercise increases the sensitivity of the body to insulin.

Dr. Philip Felig, professor of medicine at Yale University School of Medicine, reported in the *New England Journal of Medicine* that four hours of exercise per week increased insulin binding and sensitivity by 30 percent in people without diabetes. How much more effective must it be in diabetics! He concluded that exercise would improve diabetic control of blood sugar even in the absence of weight loss.[9]

Blood Pressure Control

Hypertension is a very common component of diabetes. In most studies, those with diabetes are more than twice as likely to develop high blood pressure. The side effects of the medications used to treat high blood pressure, combined with the neuropathy that comes with elevated blood sugars, makes impotence an almost certain reality for men with diabetes. That's not all.

The Sixth Report of the Joint National Committee on Prevention, Detection, Evaluation, and Treatment of High Blood Pressure concluded that the cardiovascular risks from hypertension were greatly exaggerated when diabetes was also present. They concluded that the control of blood pressure is even more important than tight blood sugar control to prevent heart attacks and strokes.

The role of exercise as an effective tool for the management of hypertension is well established. Additionally, although there are no studies to date that examine whether or not regular exercise prevents hypertension, the odds are good that it does since exercise is known to reduce blood pressure, even in those with normal readings.

Effects on Coronary Artery Disease

One of the most common complications of diabetes is coronary artery disease (CAD). Not only does regular exercise prevent CAD, it's also an effective treatment for it. Exercise has been shown to improve blood flow in diabetic patients with CAD, even when the degree of plaque obstruction remains the same. This is so for several reasons.

First, exercise reverses the age-related decrease in the ability of the heart to fill up with blood, called left ventricular diastolic function. This decrease is often seen in diabetics.

Second, exercise restores the impaired endothelial function that is also commonly seen in both diabetes and prediabetes. The endothelial cells are those cells that make up the blood vessels that go to the heart, and when their function is impaired, they constrict, thereby decreasing blood flow. Endothelial dysfunction is a major factor in heart attacks and sudden death.

Last, exercise improves blood flow by decreasing blood viscosity, or thickness. When the blood is thicker, it is less able to flow through the small capillaries and the result is decreased flow. This kind of blockage is thought to be at the center of why those with diabetes are so prone to kidney failure and blindness. The blood of patients with diabetes is on average about 8 percent more viscous than nondiabetics. Exactly why this is so remains unclear, but it is apparent that decreased levels of testosterone play a significant role, and one of those roles probably has to do with fibrinogen.

Increased blood fibrinogen levels are one of the indicators of thick blood, and increased blood fibrinogen is commonly found in those with diabetes. Administration of testosterone decreases these levels so consistently that I am now of the opinion that elevated fibrinogen levels are simply an indicator of the need for testosterone.

But we are talking about exercise here, and I want to be sure to tell you that exercise has been shown to improve impaired blood flow characteristics by as much as 30 percent.

EXERCISE VERSUS WORK

For some strange reason, Americans are troubled by the idea of exercising. This is so often the case that I have come to believe that we have some kind of unconscious primitive belief system that tells us that we need to conserve our energy so as to avoid "unnecessary" exertion at all costs. Therefore, as I see it, in order to obey this belief system we are forced to come up with a constant stream of excuses for why we can't exercise.

The most common excuse is "I don't have the time," and running a close second is the all-too-familiar "I don't have the energy." Of course, this last one is particularly ironic because exercise is extremely effective at increasing energy production.

The third most common category of exercise-avoidance excuses is the work excuse. This comes in several versions, such as "But I work in my garden," "My job is physical," "I have stairs in my house," "I play golf," or my favorite, "My wife and I go shopping a lot." As you can imagine, I've heard them all. I have no doubt that these activities require some level of exertion and are helpful in many ways, but they do not in any way substitute for a regular exercise program. Here's why.

A regular exercise program is just that. First, it is *regular*, meaning that it occurs at regular intervals such as once a day or three times a week. Second, it is *exercise*, which means that it is a controlled process that induces both maximal aerobic capacity and maximal fat metabolism. Daily activities such as the ones mentioned above that are just part of our everyday life are not able to meet this criteria in any kind of consistent way.

Last, it is a *program*, which means that a particular protocol is followed. As you will see toward the end of this chapter, my work with Bio-Energy Testing has shown me that the most effective protocol for exercise is "interval training," using the heart rate information that is provided by Bio-Energy Testing. The daily activities of your life are fun and I'm glad you enjoy them, but they are just not able to meet any of the criteria of a regular exercise program, and therefore cannot be used as a substitute.

WHAT HAPPENS WHEN YOU EXERCISE?

While you sit in your chair reading this book, if you have the kind of metabolism that I would like you to have, your body is efficiently burning fat to meet just about all of your energy needs. When, however, you become so inspired by reading this chapter that you immediately put down the book and begin exercising, your body will begin to do two things. First, it will produce more energy, which is exactly what we want it to do. Second, it will burn more fat to provide this increase in energy. That's even better.

Now, as you realize how much fun you are having and you begin to steadily increase your level of exertion, you will be increasing both your energy production and your fat metabolism. These increases will continue until you arrive at a level of exertion that is so high that your body will not be able to meet your energy needs from fat alone. On Bio-Energy Testing, this point is the point at which your heart rate equals your FBR (fat-burning heart rate; see Chapter 2).

At that point, your body will be burning the maximum amount of fat. Of course, if you are really healthy and fit, your fat-burning capability will be optimal and you will be working quite hard at this point. Conversely, to the degree that the effects of aging, hormonal deficiency, poor diet, lack of sleep, and so on, are robbing you of energy, you will hardly be exerting much energy at all when you reach your FBR.

As you continue to increase your exercise intensity above your maximum level of fat metabolism, you will steadily increase your energy output, which is good, but you will also steadily decrease the proportion of energy that is coming from fat. Ultimately, as you continue in this fashion, you will find yourself exercising at a level at which you are no longer able to derive any of your energy needs from fat, and all your energy will be created from blood sugar. On Bio-Energy Testing, this is the point at which your heart rate equals your ATR (anaerobic threshold heart rate), where you reach your maximum aerobic workout. If you will remember from Chapter 2, exercising beyond this point for any sustained period of time is damaging to your health because it forces you to enter into anaerobic metabolism.

So you can see that depending on how you exercise, you are burning maximal amounts of fat, burning no fat at all, obtaining a maximal aerobic workout, or damaging your health. When performed correctly, exercise results in improved overall energy production combined with improved fat metabolism, which is exactly the correct prescription for energy deficit disorders such as diabetes and prediabetes.

By the way, while all this metabolic stuff is going on, there are several other important effects of exercise that should be mentioned. One, since the heart is a muscle, and you are making this muscle work harder, you are strengthening it. This results in a rather dramatic improvement in cardiac function. The same principle applies to the lungs and the blood vessels. Additionally, the function of the entire circulatory system is enhanced by exercise. In fact, every single physiological system in the body that influences energy production is stimulated and improved by a proper exercise protocol.

EXERCISING TOO HARD TO BE HEALTHY?

Many people, especially those who find it hard to control their weight, are actually exercising too hard for their level of fitness and genetic makeup. Often they rely on calculated heart-rate formulas that are inaccurate for thin people and way off for those who are overweight. If you calculate where your exercise level should be using these standard formulas, you are probably wasting much if not *all* of your effort.

The reason? These formulas are all based solely on age and fail to take your genes, body build, and level of fitness into consideration. Currently, the most widely used formulas by exercise experts to compute an individual's FBR and ATR are as follows:

$$FBR = 0.65 \times (220 - age)$$

$$ATR = 0.80 \times (220 - age)$$

If you've been studying up on exercise, you've probably seen these formulas or ones very similar to them in exercise books or magazines.

Note that 220 − age is a way to estimate a person's maximum heart rate, but it is an almost completely useless calculation. The potential for inaccuracy is exemplified by the fact that an overweight man with a sedentary lifestyle who was born in 1971 will come out to have the same maximum heart rate as Tour de France champion Lance Armstrong. This is extremely unlikely! The calculations get even more unrealistic when the arbitrary use of 65 percent of this erroneous maximum heart rate is somehow supposed to represent a universal FBR, and 85 percent to represent a universal ATR.

Not too long ago I published a study entitled "Is Your Patient Exercising Too Hard to Be Healthy?" (see Appendix B for more information), in which I used Bio-Energy Testing to determine the optimum exercise levels for a random group of twenty people. Basically, what the study shows is that the exercise recommendations based on the formulas given above are useless at best, and for the most part are actually dangerous. This is an important finding not least of all because fitness instructors as well as physicians commonly give such recommendations to their clients or patients.

I just recently read a chapter on exercise from a book about "being healthy and feeling younger." In this recently published bestseller, the author persisted on repeating the same old hackneyed formulas for exercise mentioned above. Applying the results of my study, 90 percent of the readers of this bestseller who follow the author's instructions will exercise at a level of exertion that will be way too much for them.

I am convinced that the primary reason that so many people in this country are adverse to exercise is that they have been subjected to these formulas and are exercising at levels that are way above their capacity. Even though they are not aware of all the biochemical and physiological reasons why exercising too hard is bad for them, people somehow intuitively know when they are doing something that is harmful, and harmful levels of exercise are no exception. Exercising too hard doesn't feel good, and they don't feel better as a result of doing it. So, naturally, they stop. To avoid this frustrating problem, let's take a look at the right way to exercise for your health.

EXERCISING SMART

The only way to really be sure you are exercising correctly, that is, neither underdoing nor overdoing it, is to have yourself analyzed with Bio-Energy Testing and determine your optimum exercise zone. As explained in Chapter 2, the optimum exercise zone is the heart-rate range bound on one end by your FBR and on the other end by your ATR. See Appendix A for a toll-free telephone number and a website that you can use to find a testing facility in your area.

But let's suppose you don't have a Bio-Energy Testing center close to you: how can you make sure that you are not hurting yourself while trying to help yourself? A good clue is breathlessness, since most people start to become breathless when they approach their ATR. Therefore, the recommendation is to exercise at a rate just below the point where you become breathless. Let's say you're on the treadmill. You gradually increase your speed. At some point, you will start huffing and puffing, at which time you should look at your heart rate monitor. The reading will be close to your ATR. Multiply this estimated ATR by 0.60 to guesstimate your FBR.

Interval Training

There are two forms of exercise, and both of them are important for diabetics. The first form is known as interval training. This involves alternating intervals of time at your FBR with intervals at your ATR.

A typical interval-training session goes like this: First, be sure to strap on your heart rate monitor so you can keep track of your heart rate while you exercise. Begin by exercising hard enough to raise your heart rate up to your FBR. Then, after four minutes at your FBR, start exercising hard enough to bring your heart rate up to your ATR, and leave it there for one minute. Then decrease the intensity of exercise so that your heart rate comes down to your FBR. Exercise at your FBR for four minutes again, and then go back to exercising at your ATR for another minute. Continue repeating the cycle of four minutes of FBR followed by one minute of ATR for a thirty- to forty-minute exercise period.

Anaerobic Burst

Remember when I told you that any sustained exercise above your ATR is counterproductive and outright unhealthy? Well the byword here is "sustained". Because as it turns out, brief bursts of exercise above your ATR are actually very beneficial. They increase your overall maximum energy production by stretching your mitochondrial function, and they are also powerful stimulants to your anti-oxidant buffering enzymes.

So while you are engaging in the interval training I just discussed, about every eight to ten minutes I want you to go as hard and as fast as you can, and drive your heart rate much higher than your ATR for somewhere between 30-60 seconds. This brief anaerobic burst will leave you quite breathless and with a strongly pumping heart, so at the end of it slow down and allow your heart rate to recover to your FBR. Once you feel good and recovered, go on and continue your interval training.

Resistance Training

The second form of exercise is called resistance training, also referred to as bodybuilding and weight training. This is an extremely effective form of exercise, and the combination of resistance training with interval training truly delivers a knockout punch to diabetes.

Resistance training involves exercising certain muscle groups to their point of exhaustion. This is accomplished using either weights or resistance machines. I recommend that my patients consult with a physical trainer familiar with this form of exercise in order to insure that their technique is correct and that they won't hurt themselves by pulling a muscle, and so on.

The basic muscle groups that need to be exercised are the shoulder, chest, back, abdominal, and leg muscles. These muscle groups can easily be exercised using the military press, bench press, pull-down or rows, abdominal crunches, and leg squats. I recommend that each muscle group be exercised seven to ten times (this is referred to as seven to ten repetitions), being sure to adjust the weight or resistance so that you can just barely finish the last repetition.

I tell my patients to perform these exercises as though they were in a slow-motion movie, taking about five to seven seconds to push the weight up, and another five to seven seconds to bring it back to position. This slow-motion action serves two purposes: First, it prevents any muscle strains or injuries caused by rapid, jerky movements. Second, because the muscle is under tension for a longer period of time, the slow motion results in a much better training effect on the muscle.

As in interval training, make sure that you put on your heart rate monitor. After each series of repetitions (referred to as a "set"), you will notice that your heart rate is high, often higher than your ATR. If it is, this means that your metabolism became anaerobic for a few seconds, and although by now you must know that sustained exercise above your ATR is unhealthy, short bursts into this zone as discussed above are actually very beneficial because they stimulate your liver to clear lactic acid from your body more efficiently. If your heart rate is not greater than your ATR, go on to the next set. If it is, sit down and read the newspaper until your heart rate has returned to your FBR before you go on to perform another set of repetitions. In this way, you will be getting the absolute maximum benefit from each one of your workouts.

Many people erroneously think that the only good form of exercise is hard and fast. That may be a great way to win a race, but it is not the best way to stay healthy. No matter whether you are interval training or resistance training, it is very important to always alternate between exercising at your FBR and exercising at your ATR. Even though it is easier than spending your entire exercise time at your ATR, this training method is much more effective than any other way. It is also healthier, not to mention more fun!

My 5–10 Rule

Those with diabetes and prediabetes need to come to terms with this fact: although there are always exceptions, on average they need to exercise at least thirty to forty minutes, six days a week. Exercise on three of those days should consist of interval training, and on the other three, resistance training. Studies have clearly shown that anything less than this will not be as effective at controlling or eliminating the disease.

But I know what it's like to be human, and how easy it is to find reasons why I can't do the things that I need to do. How many times have you arrived for your regularly scheduled exercise program only to find that you just don't feel up to it? I don't know about you, but this happens to me about 70 percent of the time. My inner voice starts rebelling: "I'm too tired," or "I just don't feel like it right now."

A long time ago I decided I had to develop a way of dealing with this rebellion in order to pursue any semblance of a regular exercise schedule. So I came up with what I call my 5–10 rule. It works for me. See if it works as well for you. It goes like this: No matter how you feel, start your exercise. No excuses. Just do it. If, after five minutes you actually feel worse than you did when you started, call it quits for the day. If you don't feel worse, however, continue for another five minutes. If after ten minutes, you don't actually feel better than you did before you started, you can also stop.

I can honestly tell you that when you use this "yardstick," you'll end up quitting only a very small percentage of the time. It just reaffirms what I see as the incredible, energizing impact of exercise on both the physical and mental level.

So, except for the fact that exercise has been shown to lower blood pressure, increase bone strength, dramatically decrease all diseases including cancer and heart disease, improve memory, increase longevity, increase quality of life, improve sex, decrease depression, and improve sleep, there really would be no good reason for taking it on. And, of course, for diabetics and diabetes prevention in particular, nothing is as important as regular exercise. It lowers blood sugar while at the same time lowering insulin levels. Shy of taking medications, nothing else you can do will accomplish both of these feats, and exercise when done correctly is a lot more fun than taking pills. And finally, after you have convinced yourself that your couch potato days are over, be sure to exercise smart instead of exercising hard. Finding your exercise zone, or sweet spot, is another one of the benefits of Bio-Energy Testing.

CHAPTER 9

STEP FOUR:
Supporting the Liver

"Health nuts are going to feel stupid someday,
lying in hospitals dying of nothing."
—REDD FOXX, COMEDIAN (1922–1991)

f I were to ask you what you considered to be the most important organ in the body, almost all of you would likely say the brain. There's no doubt the brain is critical for the coordinated function and regulation of the body, but you would be wrong to assume that it is the most important organ. Indeed, even in the face of a significant loss of brain tissue and function, it is possible for the body to survive.

I would submit to you that the most important organ in the body is the liver. I don't think it is coincidental that if you were to drop the last letter in the name of this organ, it would spell "live." Unlike the brain, when a significant amount of function is lost in the liver, the body will very quickly die, often in a matter of only days.

The liver is so important to the minute-by-minute functioning of your body that better than a third of your entire blood supply is constantly circulating through it. Proper liver function is absolutely critical for maintaining energy production, blood sugar levels, fat metabolism, hormonal balances, blood clotting, and cell membranes, just to name its primary roles.

To the degree that your liver is not functioning optimally, your body will fail in all of these essential life-sustaining areas, and you will age faster and become more likely to develop diseases such as diabetes. In fact, in those millions of people who have inherited the genes for diabetes, optimal liver function can single-handedly spell the difference between getting the disease and not getting it.

This issue is particularly important because most physicians assume that if the liver is not overtly diseased, it is working well. Unfortunately, nothing could be further from the truth. The liver is not just the most important organ in the body, it is also the most vulnerable. It is constantly being exposed to heavy levels of bacteria, parasites, and other extremely toxic metabolites that are coming from the intestines. This exposure is so striking that if only a third of the blood that comes from the intestines were somehow to bypass your liver, you would die from infection in a matter of hours. In other words, your liver is constantly saving your life.

Not only is the liver protecting you from intestinal toxicity, but it is also responsible for cleaning the blood of all the toxins that enter the body through other means, such as through the skin and lungs. When examined from this perspective, it is easy to appreciate that your liver is constantly under siege from both your internal and your external environment, and in order to bear up to this continuous attack, it needs all the help it can get.

Because of the central function that the liver plays in the availability of glucose and fat to the cells, and because of the liver's controlling effect on the thyroid and adrenal hormones, optimal liver function is essential for optimal energy production—and, therefore, critical for the prevention and management of diabetes. In fact, the liver plays such a critical role in blood sugar management that there is even a form of diabetes known as "liver diabetes mellitus," which is reviewed in a very recent article in the journal *Medical Hypothesis*.[1]

In the rest of this chapter you will learn about the intricate processes that occur in the liver that are essential to the maintenance of proper blood sugar control and fat metabolism. You will also learn how to diagnose suboptimal liver function, as well as what you can do to insure that your liver will continue to "constantly save your life."

THE LIVER AND BLOOD SUGAR CONTROL

When asked what organ is responsible for controlling blood sugar, physicians will immediately respond that it is the pancreas. After all, the pancreas establishes ultimate control by synthesizing both the hormone glucagon, which causes an elevation in blood sugar, and also insulin, which causes a decrease in blood sugar. More importantly, the role of the pancreas is so critical that when the pancreas fails, irreversible diabetes results.

Nevertheless, it is important to note the very special role played by the liver in the regulation of blood sugar. This chapter will show you just how much optimizing liver function can do to maintain optimum blood sugar control.

After you eat a meal containing carbohydrate, the carbohydrate is quickly converted into sugar by the digestive processes, and is then absorbed by the intestines. This, of course, would immediately lead to an elevation of the blood sugar were the liver not to exert its effects. But the liver plays a central role in regulating just how high and fast the blood sugar rises, as well as how long it stays elevated.

Remember that the blood coming from the intestines, which contains all the nutrients, sugars, and so on from your meal, first passes through the liver before it can enter the general circulation. As it passes through the liver, the liver immediately acts to lower the sugar levels by converting the sugar into two storage molecules. This function of the liver is referred to as its "glucose buffer function."

One of these storage molecules is called glycogen. Glycogen serves as a quickly available, short-term form of glucose storage. When immediate energy is needed, it is glycogen that can be instantly broken down into glucose.

The other storage molecule is an energy fat called triglyceride. Virtually all of the triglyceride formation from dietary carbohydrates that occurs in the body happens in the liver. Each triglyceride molecule is a combination of two fat molecules united by a molecule called glycerol.

Triglycerides represent a long-term form of glucose storage. Some of the triglyceride molecules are stored in the liver and the rest are released into the bloodstream and eventually end up being stored in your fat cells. In these two places, triglycerides are readily available on an as-needed basis to be used to supply all your everyday nonemergency energy needs.

It is these actions of the liver that determine, to a large extent, how elevated your blood sugar is at any one time. Your liver's capacity for glycogen and triglyceride formation and storage, as well as the speed at which it can perform these functions is directly related to its overall operating efficiency. Provided that you don't eat more carbohydrate than is right for you, and provided that your liver is optimally functioning, the rise in blood sugar after you eat will be almost negligible.

Exactly how much your blood sugar rises after eating is best determined by measuring your hemoglobin A1c. Many of my diabetic patients who find it hard to control their hemoglobin A1c levels find that by simply adjusting their carbohydrate intake to the capacity of their livers, along with taking the measures to improve liver function described in this chapter, they are able to have hemoglobin A1c levels below 5.5 percent. Levels below 5.5 percent are essentially nondiabetic levels and represent perfect blood sugar control.

Many patients with diabetes swing from an elevated blood sugar to an abnormally low blood sugar, a condition that can be life threatening. When this becomes a common occurrence, the patient is often said to have "brittle diabetes." Brittle diabetes simply refers to a diabetic's condition when his liver has ceased to optimally function. There are two ways that an optimally functioning liver can prevent the low blood sugars typical of brittle diabetes.

Glucose and Glycogen

The first way the liver can prevent low blood sugar is by releasing glucose from glycogen stores when the blood sugar starts to fall as a result of the increased energy demands of exercise or stress. This is the preferred way of dealing with emergency needs for glucose, because glycogen can be converted into glucose almost immediately.

One of the problems you can encounter on the road to diabetes is that as a result of your body making the switch from primarily metabolizing fat to glucose metabolism (as described in Part I), it is likely that your increased dependency on glucose has already depleted your glycogen stores, and has in so doing set you up for those sudden episodes of low blood sugar so characteristic of brittle diabetes. In this case, it will be imperative for you to take all the measures described in this book to return your body to optimal fat metabolism, and thus allow your liver to maintain a consistent supply of glycogen.

A highly functioning liver is able to replenish glycogen stores continuously, even as they are exploited throughout the day for your various energy needs. The process responsible for this is gluconeogenesis. Gluconeogenesis refers to the conversion in the liver of protein molecules into glycogen. Since cortisol is so instrumental to gluconeogenesis, a combination of both cortisol deficiency along with a diet deficient in protein will impair gluconeogenesis, causing glycogen stores to become depleted and brittle diabetes to result. This is one of the primary reasons why it is so fundamental for diabetics to treat any underlying cortisol deficiency, and to have a diet rich in protein. (For more information on cortisol, please see Chapter 12.)

In addition to activating gluconeogenesis, the highly functioning liver also has the capability of breaking down its stored triglyceride molecules into their two components, fats and glycerol. The glycerol is then further converted to glycogen, thus providing the liver with yet another way to maintain its critical glycogen stores. Both of these metabolic activities insure that low glucose levels and brittle diabetes will not occur in a patient with optimal liver function.

Fats to the Rescue

The second way your liver can prevent low blood sugar is by providing the bloodstream with a continuous supply of fats. This insures that your cells have adequate fat available for energy production, and therefore do not have to rely on glucose metabolism, thereby preserving your glycogen stores. It works like this.

As I described, to fulfill your body's daily energy requirements, the liver busily maintains your glycogen stores through the process of gluco-neogenesis as well as by breaking down its stored triglycerides into fats and glycerol. While the glycerol then goes on to be converted to glycogen, the fats are further processed by the liver into a more easily transportable form of fat called acetoacetate. The acetoacetate is then released into the bloodstream where it can be delivered to your cells to be converted into energy. Presto! Two birds are killed with one stone—glycogen from the glycerol and then fat from the acetoacetate. Don't tell me this system isn't absolutely remarkable!

Please keep in mind that all these processes are completely dependent on how well your liver is able to function. Am I doing a good job so far in convincing you that your liver is pretty important for adequate blood sugar control?

THE LIVER AND PROTEIN SYNTHESIS

As we have seen, diabetes is an energy deficit disorder, and anything that causes decreased energy production will aggravate diabetes. One of the key elements in the production of energy in the human body takes place in a biochemical cycle that occurs in each and every cell—the citric acid cycle.

It sounds very technical and it is, but the basics are really quite simple. Let me explain.

Water (H_2O) is a molecule consisting of two hydrogen atoms combined with one oxygen atom. It has the lowest energy potential of any molecule on earth. Oxygen, on the other hand, is the highest-energy molecule on the planet. Therefore, when your body adds two hydrogen molecules to an oxygen atom, making water, it is converting the highest energy molecule in the world to the lowest. When it does this, the net energy difference is released to power every single aspect of your being, and you get to stay alive.

The citric acid cycle is what provides the hydrogen atoms that are ultimately combined with oxygen to form water in this energy-producing process called life. The citric acid cycle (also known as the Krebs cycle and the tricarboxylic cycle) is a series of biochemical reactions that occurs in the mitochondria. Fats and glucose enter into this cycle and through a number of steps are relieved of their hydrogen content.

Now that you can see why the citric acid cycle is so essential to life, it may interest you to know that many of the key elements of the citric acid cycle are proteins that are made in the liver. To the degree that your liver may not be functioning perfectly in this regard, the entire energy production of every cell in your body becomes impaired.

Another key aspect of protein synthesis in the liver is the production of blood or plasma proteins. These proteins are essential to health and play a critical role in a number of functions. For one, they serve as important pH buffers. This means that they are able to protect your body from the effects of the acids formed during energy production. Another important function of these proteins is that they maintain normal blood volume by preventing all the fluid in your blood from diffusing out into your tissues and turning you into a soggy bog.

Additionally, almost all of your hormones are attached to plasma proteins. In Chapter 6, we discussed SHBG, a protein that binds up testosterone. This attachment, called protein binding, prevents your hormones from being lost in your urine. A deficiency of these plasma proteins would result in a deficiency of virtually every hormone in your body. SHBG and all the other binding proteins are formed in the liver when the liver is stimulated by thyroid hormone.

And finally, because plasma proteins also serve as carrier molecules for metals, minerals, fats, amino acids, enzymes, and even medications, a shortage results in a significant impairment in the function of every organ in your body. Every single one of these plasma proteins are made in your liver.

IT GOES ON AND ON AND ON . . .

I could go on and on (maybe you're thinking I already have) about all the marvelous functions of the liver. Among them:

- The liver is responsible for converting T4, the inactive form of thyroid hormone, to T3, the active form. It does this on an as-needed basis, but to the degree that the liver doesn't perform this conversion very well, hypothyroidism will develop. (We will discuss thyroid hormones in more detail in Chapter 12.)

- Virtually every vitamin and mineral that you take into your body must first be processed by the liver before it can be of any use to your cells.

- The liver insures adequate blood levels of many critical vitamins and minerals as vitamin A, vitamin D, vitamin B_{12}, and iron by providing large storage compartments for these nutrients.

- All of your adrenal and sex hormones are made from the cholesterol that your liver makes, and even the very cell membranes of every cell in your body are dependent on the liver producing enough phospholipids for cell membrane function. Keep all this in mind when you remember how important cell membranes are for the function of insulin and other important hormones in the treatment of diabetes.

TESTING LIVER FUNCTION

Unfortunately, as I mentioned before, most physicians don't really take liver function into consideration unless the liver is diseased. Part of the reason for this is that there are really very few ways available to assess how optimally a person's liver is functioning. For example, if your liver-function blood tests come back as normal, it doesn't mean that your liver is healthy, it just means that it isn't diseased. The same is true with results of a liver scan.

Of course, if your diabetes is well controlled as indicated by a hemoglobin A1c level below 5.5 percent, and if you are not having any episodes of low blood sugar, that alone is evidence that your liver is functioning pretty well. If this is not the case, however, there are three methods that

I use to give me an idea of how well my patient's liver is functioning.

The first is to look at the levels of a plasma protein called albumin. Albumin is the most abundant protein in the blood, its levels can be easily and inexpensively determined, and because it is entirely made in the liver, it can serve as a good indicator of liver function. The "normal" range for albumin is between 3.5 and 5 grams per deciliter (g/dl), however, optimum levels should be over 4.5 g/dl. Levels below 4.5 g/dl are often an indicator of suboptimal liver function. Whether or not a level less than 4.5 g/dl is really indicating decreased liver function can be verified by taking measures to improve function and repeating the test to see if the levels improved.

Another excellent way to assess liver function is by examining a living specimen of the patient's blood under a darkfield microscope. This has to be done immediately after obtaining the blood from a finger stick, and in my opinion should always be performed by the examining physician during any comprehensive examination. Unfortunately, however, this technique is not taught in medical schools and only a handful of physicians know about it and use it regularly.

A darkfield microscope is a special microscope that allows a physician to examine components of the blood that are not easy to see using a regular microscope. This is a remarkably sensitive way to evaluate the condition of the blood, and a physician trained in this technique is often able to detect findings that are typical of decreased liver function. Conversely, when the darkfield examination of the blood is normal, the odds are extremely good that the liver is functioning perfectly.

Finally, the third way to assess liver function is simply by using Bio-Energy Testing to assess the patient's energy production. Since the liver is so critical to the overall energy production of the body, a decrease in its functioning will often be reflected by a decrease in energy production.

HELPING YOUR LIVER

Remember that your liver is in a very vulnerable position. It is charged with detoxifying every aspect of your body. The liver both processes the incredible levels of internal toxins produced in the intestines and protects the body against the ever-increasing toxin burden from our environment. In the course of removing these toxins from the body, the liver generates an enormous amount of those dangerous molecules called free radicals. As you'll recall from Chapter 1, free radicals are normal byproducts of metabolism, but at the same time, they are highly damaging to the cells. It is universally agreed that free-radical damage is the major cause of deterioration of our bodies as we get older.

The Critical Role of Antioxidants

In order to limit the damaging effect of free radicals, Nature has evolved a variety of protective processes collectively referred to as antioxidant buffering systems. These antioxidant systems are able to attach electrons to the free-radical molecules, and in so doing, render them harmless.

There are several important nutrients that serve to protect and assist these antioxidant buffering systems, and these are referred to as antioxidants. In the absence of optimal levels of antioxidant nutrients, the antioxidant buffering systems will become overwhelmed, and increased damage from free radicals will occur. In the liver, this translates to a significant decrease in its ability to detoxify the body, and thus the liver has an enormous need for these antioxidant nutrients in order to perform optimally. The liver sucks antioxidants up like a dry sponge on a pool of water.

The primary antioxidant nutrients for the liver are vitamins C and E, lipoic acid, the amino acid glutathione, and the minerals selenium, manganese, copper, and zinc. Everybody knows about vitamins C and E. Because they are vitamins, they cannot be made in the body and therefore must be taken in through the diet. However, due to the dramatically increased exposure that we all now have to toxins from the environment, it is impossible for the liver to get enough of them from food alone, so they must be supplemented for optimum effect.

Lipoic acid, on the other hand, is already made in the body. As children, our livers and every one of our cells produced large quantities of lipoic acid. But as we get older, we manufacture less and less lipoic acid, and so it, too, must be supplemented.

Glutathione, when it is activated by the mineral selenium, forms the central component of one of the two key antioxidant enzymes in the body, glutathione peroxidase. Glutathione also can be taken in the diet but it is not absorbed very well. Instead, there is an amino acid called N-acetyl-cysteine, which when taken in the diet, is converted by the liver into glutathione.

The minerals zinc, manganese, and copper are all essential to the functioning of the other key antioxidant enzyme, superoxide dismutase.

Superoxide dismutase binds up what is considered to be the most toxic element of oxygen metabolism, the superoxide radical.

Superoxide radical is an essential part of the energy-generating systems in the body, but it must be controlled by superoxide dismutase, because if it isn't, it will permanently destroy many of the most vital components of the mitochondria and other cellular structures. Genetic damage to our very RNA and DNA primarily occurs as a result of excessive superoxide radical.

In order for superoxide dismutase to control superoxide radical it must contain zinc, copper, and manganese. As was discussed in Chapter 7, manganese is a mineral that has been found to be deficient in up to 50 percent of diabetics tested. Similarly, copper and zinc have also been found to be deficient.[2]

Deficiencies of these nutrients, as well as many others, occur as a result of several documented factors, including decreased levels in soil, poor eating habits, and decreased levels as a result of food processing.[3] An additional problem for diabetics is that they require and overutilize these nutrients to such a point that deficiencies are almost bound to happen unless the nutrients are supplemented.

Collectively, it is the amount of all of these nutrients that will determine to a large extent how well your liver functions, in addition to how resistant your body is to the ravages of disease and aging in general. It is important to note that in the process of protecting and assisting the liver, these nutrients are rapidly used up and must be replaced on a regular basis. I believe so strongly in the importance of these nutrients that I routinely prescribe them to every patient in my practice regardless of age or condition. In diabetics, these nutrients are absolutely essential to success.

The Protective Aspects of Glycogen

As I mentioned before, glycogen is the storage molecule that the liver makes from glucose and protein. It turns out that the levels of glycogen in the liver are extremely important to the detoxifying function of the liver. The chemical processes the liver uses to remove toxins from the body progress at a more efficient rate when the glycogen content of the liver is high.

A glycogen-rich liver, therefore, is much more resistant to toxic agents and pathological mechanisms. It is important to maintain optimal glycogen stores by making sure that your body is metabolizing fat efficiently, and by insuring you have an adequate amount of protein in your diet.

The Importance of Dietary Fiber

Many of the toxins that the liver removes from the body are eliminated through the bowels. In this process, the liver binds the toxic materials to bile and then excretes the bile, which then moves into the intestines. Unfortunately, it is possible that unless they are rapidly eliminated in a bowel movement, a portion of these toxic bile salts will become reabsorbed from the intestines and go right back to the liver, requiring it to go through the whole process again.

An inactivity of the bowels as is manifested by the symptom of constipation virtually assures that this will happen, and should be taken quite seriously. The presence in your diet of soluble fiber, the kind of fiber you get from vegetables and seeds—not the kind you get from grains—serves two important functions in this regard.

One, soluble fiber is able to absorb the bile salts in the intestines and thus prevent them from being returned to the liver. Second, soluble fiber provides bulk to the bowels, which promotes regular bowel movements. Ideally, your diet should have at least 25 grams of soluble fiber per day. This amount can easily be obtained by eating sufficient amounts of vegetables.

Eating Optimal Amounts

There are two basic mistakes that almost all Americans make every day when they eat. One you already know about: they eat way too much carbohydrate—so much so that even people who are on low-carbohydrate diets are still in excess. The other mistake is that Americans eat way too much in general. We love our food, and anything we love we want more of. And unfortunately, in this country it is all too easy to get "supersized." In fact, most portions in America are already supersized, whether they are called that or not.

When you are young, due to the high metabolic activity associated with growing, it is often easy to get away with eating a lot more than you really need. I think it is in these years that we acquire the bad habit of overeating, and somehow we develop the unconscious opinion that eating until we are stuffed is the way to go. It also doesn't help that in the very first years of our lives we are constantly admonished to "Eat, eat" or "Finish your _____ (meat, vegetables, bread, and so on)."

At any rate, no matter what your theory is, I think you will agree with me that many of us, skinny and fat alike, eat a lot more than we need to.

Besides all of the health implications of overeating, did you know that it is also a surefire way to damage the liver? Overeating promotes the development of a condition called hepatosteatosis, or "fatty liver" in normal language. Hepatosteatosis is more common than many of us would like to think, and it is present in just about anybody who chronically overeats.

So, instead of supersizing your liver by overeating, how about supersizing your health and your enjoyment of life by eating only as much as you need to? In this country, that's hard but it can be done if you make a point of it.

Dr. Shallenberger's Super Immune QuickStart-DM

A long time ago I realized, like I hope you do too, that the function of the liver was centrally important to health. I decided to do everything I could to make it easy for my patients to help their livers function at a high level. So, in addition to educating them about how to take better care of their liver through a proper lifestyle, I also developed a comprehensive nutritional supplement that I ended up calling QuickStart.

I put a lot of thought and research, and twenty-five years of experience with patients into the formulation of this unique blend of nutrients, herbs, and amino acids, and it has really paid off. My patients routinely report improvements in just about every area of biological function that you can imagine. Why? Because QuickStart was formulated with optimum liver function in mind.

Subsequently, my research into the causes of diabetes led me to add key ingredients for glucose control to form a special version of QuickStart designed for those with diabetes. This supplement is called QuickStart-DM. While it has never been meant to be a substitution for a healthy diet, the spectrum and doses of QuickStart-DM are state of the art in the nutritional management of diabetes.

I did not write this book to sell QuickStart-DM. I created the formula long before I wrote this book, to fill a vacuum. I wanted to save my patients the money and time required to take all of the ingredients separately. And there just wasn't anything on the market that met my criteria. I don't really care if you buy QuickStart-DM or simply take all the ingredients found in it in a separate form. In fact, in case you want to do that, I have included in Appendix A all the ingredients along with their correct doses. If you decide to take a substitute, that's okay, too. As long as you and your physician are happy, I'm happy.

QuickStart-DM comes in powder form. I tell patients to use it, along with another product called Super Fat. These two products can be blended along with some ice, yogurt, and/or protein powder to create a great-tasting "power breakfast" smoothie that literally gives them a rocket boost each morning. (Appendix A also provides a listing of ingredients in Super Fat.) Because it is designed to powerfully assist the activity of the liver, QuickStart-DM has all of the antioxidant nutrients mentioned in the discussion of antioxidants above, as well as all the cofactors the liver requires to perform its many important roles. In addition, it has therapeutic support for increasing fat metabolism and insulin sensitivity.

QuickStart-DM is formulated to do the following:

- Increase energy production

- Improve fat metabolism

- Improve insulin sensitivity

- Stabilize blood sugars

- Maximize liver function and detoxification

- Alkalinize tissues

- Improve circulation

- Stabilize the appetite

- Enhance immunity

- Provide complete nutritional and antioxidant protection

- Remove heavy metals

It is important to mention that QuickStart-DM is unlike the great majority of combination products out there. It does not contain meaningless doses of many nutrients just to make the label look good. Every ingredient is tried and true, and is added in its *full therapeutic dose.* As a consequence, it's a little bit more expensive than other products, but worth it. Compare labels before you compare prices. See Appendix A for information about purchasing QuickStart-DM, as well as Super Fat. If you decide you would rather take the contents of QS-DM in separate supplements, just make sure that you take all of the ingredients in the recommended doses, and your liver will be thanking you for a long time.

CHAPTER 10

STEP FIVE:
Sleep

I have never taken any exercise except sleeping and resting.
—MARK TWAIN, WRITER, HUMORIST (1835–1910)

This quip from Mark Twain is funny because it plays on the commonly held belief that sleep is just a period of unproductive, wasted time, that nothing really important happens during sleep. I hope this chapter will convince you that nothing could be further from the truth.

"Get plenty of sleep" is the age-old physician's prescription for recuperating, but it's also a prescription for staying healthy. And today, even in this modern age of medical marvels, getting enough high-quality sleep is as important as ever. Yet I find that adequate sleep is a challenge for many patients. As you already know, there are many aspects of our stress-oriented, 24/7 lifestyles that don't do a lot to help us stay healthy. Not getting enough sleep is a good example of this. In fact, many of us knowingly or otherwise have actually adopted the attitude that "if you snooze you lose."

I often meet people who brag about how little sleep they need. They see it as a sign of strength. "I can get by on only four to five hours of sleep and still exercise and have a fully productive day," they'll say. Bertrand Russell who won the Nobel Prize for literature in 1950 once said, "Men who are unhappy, like men who sleep badly, are always proud of the fact." This macho attitude may impress some of their friends, but I see it more as an act of self-destruction. These people have no idea how negatively they are impacting their health by avoiding sleep.

In the 1950s, the American Cancer Society conducted a very large study to try to determine the major lifestyle factors that caused cancer and decreased life span in general. The study examined sleep habits as well as smoking, diet, cholesterol levels, blood pressure, exercise, and so on. Over 1 million Americans were surveyed over a six-year period, and the habits of those who died during this space of time were identified. Out of all the factors studied, the amount of sleep time was the best predictor of mortality. The highest death rates for all ages were for those who slept four hours or less per night, and the lowest rates were for those who regularly slept eight hours.

Other investigators have published studies revealing similar outcomes. One study in particular looked at 1,600 adults between the ages of thirty-six and fifty and found that compared with good sleepers, poor sleepers were 6.5 times more likely to have any one of a variety of health problems.

William Dement, M.D., Ph.D., is the founder and director of the Stanford University Sleep Research Center and one of the original pioneers in the study of sleep, and the lack of it. The back of Dr. Dement's excellent book, *The Promise of Sleep*, states, "Healthful sleep has been empirically proven to be the single most important factor in predicting longevity, more influential than diet, exercise, or heredity. And yet we are a sleep-sick society, ignorant of the facts of sleep and the price of sleep deprivation." Dr. Dement underlines this point even more when he states, "From the perspective of longevity, sleep may turn out to be more important than most people think. There is plenty of compelling evidence supporting the argument that sleep is the most important predictor of how long you will live, perhaps more important than whether you smoke, exercise, or have high blood pressure or cholesterol levels."[1]

If you consider that one of your jobs is to do whatever it takes to be healthy, then it's time to start sleeping on the job. The English playwright Thomas Dekker stated over 300 years ago, "Sleep is the golden chain that ties health and our bodies together." I often wonder if we have learned as much about health in the last 300 years as he knew then. My own observation over the last thirty years of doctoring my patients has been that those patients who sleep the best also feel the best, and usually have the healthiest results on Bio-Energy Testing.

According to a 1997 article in the *New York Times Magazine*, many sleep researchers believe that sleep deprivation is reaching "crisis proportions." This is a problem not just for serious insomniacs, but for the population at large, the article said, adding, "People don't merely believe they're sleeping less; they are *in fact* sleeping less—perhaps as much as one and a half hours less each night than humans did at the beginning of the century—often because they choose to do so."[2]

Many of us have gotten into the habit of going to bed late in order to read, to watch late-night TV, or to catch up on some other activity that we don't find enough time for during the day. Sleep deprivation is just a bad habit like any other. I am constantly reminding my patients how important sleep really is, and that not getting enough of it can be a major barrier to their health. This is particularly true when it comes to the treatment and prevention of diabetes.

And the attitude of catching up on lost sleep "when I have the time" just doesn't cut it. Without adequate sleep your fat metabolism is derailed and your energy production subsequently falls to very unhealthy levels. Sleep deprivation, whether out of choice or because of insomnia, shortens your life and increases the likelihood of a whole variety of diseases, including cancer, obesity, and of course diabetes.

YOUR TWO-PHASE BODY

Perhaps Dr. Allan Rechtschaffen, a well-respected sleep researcher at the University of Chicago said it best, "If sleep does not serve an absolutely vital function, then it is the biggest mistake the evolutionary process has ever made."[3] So what is this absolutely vital function that sleep offers us?

Your body runs basically on two twelve-hour phases. The time between 6:00 A.M. and 6:00 P.M. is called the "catabolic" phase. During this phase, your body is willing to do pretty much anything to keep you up and running. That means it is going to continually rob Peter to pay Paul. Simplistically speaking, if your left leg needs something that your right leg has, your body will borrow it from the right leg and give it to the left. If your heart needs some raw material more urgently than your adrenal glands, the body will make sure that your heart gets it, and your adrenal glands will have to make do. This process is called catabolism, and it results in damage to certain tissues in order to keep others with a higher priority running efficiently.

But don't worry. Your body is quite smart. Enter phase two: the "anabolic" phase. This is the time when the body repairs all the damage and "borrowing" that went on during the catabolic phase. The body's repair hours are between 6:00 P.M. and 6:00 A.M., and we call the process "anabolism." Anabolism takes place while we are sleeping (or should be).

This is a key point. The body repairs damage through the medium of rather subtle energy fields that cannot be effective during the active part of the day. These fields organize the repair effort and reach their maximum potential during sleep, particularly the deeper levels of sleep.

The maintenance of the anabolic phase during sleep is precisely why sleep is so important. Without an adequate sleep period, we are unable to fully repair the damage we create during the day. This is also why sleep is even more important to those who exercise and lead very active lives. A chronic lack of adequate sleep results in an accelerated deterioration of the body due to the accumulated damage that was never adequately repaired, thus leading us down the path to premature aging, disease, and diabetes.

BRAIN FUNCTION AND THE IMMUNE SYSTEM

There are also a number of other critical processes that happen during sleep that are less understood than the catabolic-anabolic cycle. We don't quite know the details of how these other functions of sleep are actualized, but we do know that they exist, because research has observed that these functions predictably deteriorate during periods of sleep deprivation. One of the most significant of these functions has to do with the brain.

According to the Roffwarg-Dement theory, the primary purpose of stage 2 sleep, also known as REM (rapid eye movement) sleep, is brain development. In other words, in the absence of adequate sleep, the brain deteriorates. The symptoms of this effect are clearly seen in the association of sleep disorders with mental and emotional breakdowns.

Experimental studies have also demonstrated that sleep deprivation results in impairment of memory and recall. For example, in a particularly disturbing 1987 study, researchers examined the effect of sleep loss in elderly subjects and noted an association between decreased REM sleep and dementia and depression.[4] In another study on the relationship between REM sleep and Alzheimer's disease, the author states, "REM sleep deficit may explain the progression and/or the acceleration of memory loss in Alzheimer's disease."[5]

Another important area of human function vitally tied to sleep is the immune system. The hormone melatonin is secreted during sleep and is blocked from being released during the waking hours. Thus, whenever there is an insufficient amount of sleep, there is also a melatonin deficiency. Melatonin is critical for the induction of sleep, particularly REM sleep, but it is also critical for the optimum functioning of the immune system. It also has an anticancer function, and is even used to treat a variety of cancers.

Melatonin has been found to be active in the formation of both antibodies and certain immune-related compounds known as cytokines. Three of these cytokines, tumor-necrosis (necrosis means "killing") factor (TNF), interleukin-1, and interleukin-2 are produced during sleep in response to melatonin secretion. TNF, in particular, is a potent killer of cancer cells, and circulating levels of TNF are ten times greater when we are asleep than when we are awake. In other words, when I am asleep, my body is not doing nothing. The fact is that it is busy killing any fledgling cancer cells wanting to grow up and take over.

Additionally, there are several other very important hormones that are produced primarily during sleep that are particularly important in the prevention and treatment of diabetes. I will discuss these in the next section.

SLEEP AND DIABETES

Sleep deprivation results in both of the characteristics needed to establish an energy deficit disorder: decreased fat metabolism and decreased total energy production. Exactly how sleep deprivation causes these two phenomena has not been made fully clear, but it is clear that a major role can be attributed to the hormonal imbalances that occur along with inadequate sleep.

One of the primary hormones that increase fat metabolism is growth hormone. Growth hormone is secreted primarily during sleep, and its production significantly falls as a result of either a decrease in the amount of total sleep and/or slow-wave sleep. Chapter 12 contains an in-depth discussion of growth hormone, and in Chapter 14 when I discuss Dale's case, you will see how growth hormone therapy can be a very helpful part of a comprehensive therapeutic approach for diabetes.

In 1999, Eve Van Cauter, a sleep researcher at the University of Chicago, reported in the journal *Lancet* that lack of adequate sleep can create a prediabetic state in the body, which in turn can contribute to obesity. Van Cauter's suggestion came after a study in which eleven young men were allowed only four hours of sleep each night for a week. Even though these healthy young men were subjected to sleep deprivation for only a short period, in that time they developed impaired glucose tolerance, essentially a prediabetic state.[6]

Another study entitled "Effects of Sleep Deprivation and Exercise on Glucose Tolerance" gives us an idea of what happens to blood sugar control when we don't get enough sleep. The researchers examined the effect of only one period of sleep deprivation in a group of men who were sedentary and in another group of men who were exercising. Both groups demonstrated a significant decrease in insulin sensitivity, although as we would expect, there was less of a decrease in the exercising group. What is important to note here is that from this study it appears that sleep may be even more important than exercise for diabetes prevention.[7]

And we are not talking about a very significant decrease in sleep time to have these negative effects. A study published in *Diabetes Care* in 2003 looked at the effect of overall sleep time in a group of more than 70,000 nurses over a ten-year period. The results are sobering to say the least.

When the results were finally analyzed, they found a 57 percent increase in the incidence of diabetes among those nurses who were getting five hours of sleep or less. When the researchers removed the other factors that are also associated with the onset of diabetes, such as obesity and lack of exercise, they discovered that a full one-third of the cases of diabetes in these nurses could be attributed solely to too little sleep! They concluded that "sleep restriction may be an independent risk factor for developing symptomatic diabetes."[8]

SLEEP AND OBESITY

The sleep-obesity connection is troubling from all angles. For starters, because it often results in a condition called obstructive sleep apnea, obesity itself impairs sleep. Let me explain the connection.

When we sleep, we go through four stages. Each stage is a progressively deeper level of sleep. Stage 4 sleep is so deep that the body is essentially in a coma. As we get deeper into these stages, the muscles throughout the body become more and more relaxed, and this includes the muscles that keep our breathing airway open.

Obesity causes an increase in fat all over the body, including the fat in the tissues in and around our breathing airway. As these tissues become overburdened with fat content, they become swollen and heavy, and the muscles that keep the airway open while we are sleeping must work harder.

Sleep apnea, which literally means a cessation of breathing during sleep, occurs during the deeper levels of sleep when the muscles become so relaxed that they are unable to offset the swollen and fatty tissues around the airway. When this happens, the airway collapses and the patient stops breathing. This cessation of breathing can last anywhere from one to three minutes before the patient suddenly restarts breathing again with a gasping type of breath. Of course, since the patient with obstructive sleep apnea is asleep, he or she is not aware that all this is happening. However, the spouse will often report observing this kind of irregular breathing.

Besides the swelling in the airway, fat accumulation in the abdomen is also a factor in obstructive sleep apnea because the increased weight on the abdomen impairs abdominal breathing. You will learn more about abdominal breathing and how important it is in the next chapter, which discusses stress.

The single most reliable sign that airway obstruction is occurring is the cessation of breathing mentioned above. Another consistent sign is snoring. Patients who regularly snore, especially those who snore loudly, are good candidates for either having obstructive sleep apnea or for developing it. So, if you are becoming a snorer, it is time to lose some weight and prevent the condition before it develops.

Obstructive sleep apnea sets the stage for a scary, vicious cycle. Since a patient with obstructive sleep apnea stops breathing during the deeper stages of sleep, his or her body will not be able to get anywhere close to an adequate amount of deep-stage sleep. Van Cauter's research points out that two very important hormones, growth hormone and leptin, are secreted only during those deep stages of sleep. Both of these hormones are vitally important for weight control, and as patients with obstructive sleep apnea develop a deficiency of these hormones, they start to gain even more weight, which of course intensifies the obstructive sleep apnea.

Perhaps the most important hormone that can be affected by sleep deprivation is growth hormone. The levels of growth hormone can dramatically decline after only one night of inadequate sleep. For a complete discussion of growth hormone and its effects on fat-burning metabolism please refer to Chapter 12.

Leptin is a hormone that signals the body to stop eating. According to the findings of a 2004 study published in the *Annals of Internal Medicine*, when young healthy men were restricted to four hours of sleep for only two days all of them showed significant decreases in their leptin levels along with increased feelings of hunger and appetite.[9] What this means is that the low leptin levels caused by only minimal amounts of sleep debt will cause your body to crave carbohydrate even though you've had enough calories. This is certainly a bad recipe for diabetics. And keep in mind that these findings occur in young, healthy men in their early twenties. How much more of an effect will sleep deprivation have in those individuals who are older and less fit? The vicious cycle of obesity leading to obstructive sleep apnea leading to obesity is sometimes so overwhelming for a patient that unless the obstructive sleep apnea is corrected, it becomes almost impossible for that patient to ever get control of his or her weight.

WHEN IS SLEEP SLEEP?

While there is really no doubt in anyone's mind that sleep is necessary, there is still some confusion over just how much is needed. Your body doesn't just need some sleep. It needs enough sleep, and enough deep-stage or high-quality sleep. So how much is enough? The studies show that the healthiest, most long-lived individuals are those who regularly sleep eight hours per night.

So how do you know if you are getting enough sleep? To answer, we can again turn to Dr. William Dement. During his research into this question, Dr. Dement noted that when his experimental subjects were deprived of sleep, they fell asleep the next night much more quickly than usual. In fact, he noted that, overall, the less sleep they had over days and weeks of observation, the more quickly they fell asleep. This was true regardless of whether they went to sleep during the day or at night.

As a result of this observation, Dr. Dement developed what he called the multiple sleep latency test (MSLT). The test is rather simple and in a sense quite obvious, but like so many other "very obvious" things in science, they only become obvious after someone has noticed and investigated them. The MSLT involves determining the amount of time it takes an individual to fall asleep.

What the research shows is that people who are getting an optimal amount of sleep take about fifteen to twenty minutes to fall asleep. Those who are getting a less-than-optimal, but manageable, amount take less time to fall asleep, usually from ten to fifteen minutes. Those whose bodies are suffering from sleep deprivation tend to fall asleep in less than ten minutes, and those with severe sleep deficiency fall asleep in less than five minutes. When I first learned about this score, my initial reaction was one of surprise, because like most people I have always thought that falling asleep quickly was a good sign.

Of course, it must be taken into consideration that there are a number of other variables in what determines how quickly you fall asleep besides whether or not you are sleep deprived. These include stress, caffeine intake, sleep habits, and so on. Many people who have significant sleep disturbances still take a long time to fall asleep because of these factors.

Another indication of inadequate sleep is daytime sleepiness. This is particularly true if you have a history of taking naps or nodding off at meetings or in front of the TV. Again, lack of these symptoms does not necessarily rule out sleep deprivation because many people are able to overcome daytime sleepiness using stimulants and/or sheer willpower.

Finally comes the issue of depth of sleep. In other words, even though you are getting enough sleep, are you getting enough deep-stage sleep? Although this question can certainly be determined by an overnight stay in a diagnostic sleep facility, it is much harder to determine without that sophisticated level of investigation. Nonetheless, a fairly good way to assess sleep depth or quality is to notice how easily you are awakened compared with children.

I am sure that all of us who have observed kids sleeping have noticed that they are frequently difficult to waken. Even loud noises often fail to do the job. This is because children spend a much greater amount of time in the very deepest levels of sleep. If you find that even slight sounds easily wake you up throughout the night, then chances are that you are not sleeping deeply enough. Conversely, if your spouse tells you that you are difficult to wake up, you are probably in good shape.

Another indication of poor sleep quality occurs when an individual is getting eight hours of sleep, but is still experiencing signs of sleep deprivation, such as daytime sleepiness or falling asleep as soon as the head hits the pillow.

DIAGNOSING SLEEP DEFICIENCY

Whatever you do, please be sure to take your sleep time seriously. Often simply examining whether you have any of the indicators mentioned in the previous section, and to what degree, is enough to determine whether or not you are getting adequate sleep. For the most part, when sleep deficiency is apparent, it is really easy to handle the problem. The most common prescription is to go to bed earlier.

Be sure to get eight hours of good, solid, uninterrupted sleep in a fully darkened room, ideally before the sun comes up. If you can't do this, blacken out your room or use an eye mask so that it still seems dark even after the sun has risen. Light, even a little light, is enough to activate the waking centers of your brain and decrease your ability to enter into deep sleep. Lights left on in the room interfere with sleep. The production of melatonin is immediately cut off by exposure to light. This decrease of melatonin that occurs with light exposure is what causes us to awaken when the sun comes up. If you have to get up in the night for a trip to the bathroom, don't turn on the lights. Use a red-colored night-light. Red light does not seem to curtail melatonin production.

Other common solutions are to decrease alcohol and caffeine intake in general, and strictly avoid food and alcohol for three hours before bedtime. Studies have also shown that regular exercise enhances sleep quality, particularly if it is done in the late afternoon. If you routinely get up to urinate, be sure to restrict your fluids before bedtime. And last, if you are awakened during the night, do not look at the clock. This little habit that many of us have often causes the brain to keep us awake thinking about the time and how much sleep we are getting.

Chronic insomnia is a serious health problem. If you have this problem, don't "solve" it by taking drugs. Instead, treat the problem. Studies show that sleep medications interfere with the development of the deeper levels of sleep. If you are over forty-five years of age, try 0.5 to 3 milligrams of melatonin before bedtime. Certain herbs, especially valerian and chamomile, are especially helpful to induce sleep, and Chapter 7 also has some good ideas regarding sleep aids.

A discussion of stress and worry as a cause of insomnia is a whole other book, but I will leave you with one of my all-time favorite quotes, which seems to help me in this matter. Victor Hugo said the following more than 100 years ago: "Have courage for the great sorrows of life and patience for the small ones; and when you have laboriously accomplished your daily task, go to sleep in peace. God is awake." It doesn't help to worry at night. That is your special time to heal your body for the next day. Leave the rest to a higher power.

CHAPTER 11

STEP SIX:
Reducing Stress

*Life has no other discipline to impose, if we would but realize
it, than to accept life unquestioningly. Everything we shut our
eyes to, everything we run away from, everything we deny,
denigrate, or despise, serves to defeat us in the end. What
seems nasty, painful, evil, can become a source of beauty, joy,
and strength, if faced with an open mind. Every moment is a
golden one for him who has the vision to recognize it as such.*

    — HENRY MILLER, AUTHOR (1891–1980)

*I am still determined to be cheerful and happy, in whatever
situation I may be; for I have also learned from experience
that the greater part of our happiness or misery depends
upon our dispositions, and not upon our circumstances.*

—MARTHA WASHINGTON, WIFE OF GEORGE WASHINGTON (1732–1802)

After thirty years of medicine, it has become my belief that the two most important challenges to our health are:

1. The fact that there is a learned tendency in all of us to frequently create ever-increasing amounts of stress for ourselves.

2. The fact that all of this stress eventually wears us down.

Over and over again, I hear from my patients how concerned they are about all the negative factors in the environment, such as chemically contaminated food, water, and air. They worry about whether they should spend the extra money to buy organic produce, and whether or not it is safe to take an allergy pill, and so on. It's not that these aren't real concerns, but when I hear patients worrying over them, I often reflect to myself that the worry they have is probably affecting their health more negatively than the problems themselves. Stress is indeed rampant in our culture, and it is a serious factor in diabetes.

The problem with even discussing stress is that it is so predominant in our culture that it is as hard to identify as the pollution in the air. Too bad we don't have a stress meter. Then everybody could be tested for stress and then treated for it until the stress meter indicated acceptable levels. But then again that whole process would stress most people out even more. So let's not ask ourselves whether or not we are stressed. Let's just start working on decreasing it right now, because I promise you it is there.

WHAT STRESS DOES TO THE BODY

When chronically stressed, the body responds in a certain way. It really doesn't matter if the source of the stress is physical, like pain, insomnia, allergies, or infection, or if it is mental or emotional. The body will respond to it the same way in a rather predictable manner. There will be an increase in the adrenal gland's production of cortisol, the "stress hormone." Cortisol will exert its effect not only on the brain but on every cell in your body. There is no part of your body that will escape the effects of cortisol.

Your body's physiological stress response impacts diabetes in two ways. First, it enhances the conditions that lead to diabetes, and, second, it worsens many of the complications of diabetes. Let's take a look at these two effects.

Stress as a Major Factor Leading to Diabetes

As mentioned, the body's primary response to stress is to stimulate the adrenal gland to increase its production of cortisol. This increase in cortisol then leads to an increase in insulin production, since insulin is a counterbalancing hormone for cortisol. We have already seen how elevated levels of insulin ultimately result in decreased insulin sensitivity, thereby setting the table for diabetes if the genetic predisposition is there. This insulin-inducing effect of cortisol is so pronounced that there is a form of diabetes known as "adrenal diabetes," which results entirely from elevated levels of cortisol even in the absence of the genes for diabetes.

Adrenal diabetes is relatively uncommon, but the decrease in insulin sensitivity caused by chronic stress is not. One of the most common observations that physicians make when treating diabetics is that during times of stress, such as infection or physical or emotional pain, the blood sugar often becomes very difficult to control. This is due to the increase in cortisol that occurs in the body's stress response.

As I will discuss in more depth in Chapter 12, cortisol is a hormone that causes an increase in fat metabolism, whereas one of the primary effects of insulin is to block fat metabolism. When cortisol is secreted in excess, so much insulin is produced that the fat-burning effects of cortisol become overwhelmed by insulin, and fat metabolism ends up in a net decrease. This increase in cortisol with the subsequent increase in insulin can persist for years and never be discovered because most physicians never test for it. Furthermore, even when tests for adrenal function are performed, they can often fail to point out the condition. All during this time, however, the stage for diabetes, decreased insulin sensitivity combined with decreased fat metabolism, is being set.

But the increase in cortisol production, although in some cases it can coexist with diabetes, as a rule is just the forerunner of the disease. In the majority of cases, the continuous battle between insulin and cortisol is eventually won by insulin, and the adrenal gland goes into a state of exhaustion. When this happens, it can no longer put out enough cortisol to deal with all the insulin, much less our everyday stresses, and a relative state of cortisol deficiency happens.

Cortisol deficiency then further intensifies the entire imbalance because it causes a decrease in sugar stores, which leads to carbohydrate craving, an even further decrease in fat metabolism, a total decrease in energy production, and an increase in anaerobic energy production. The body goes into an energy-deficit state, and if the genes for diabetes are already there, the patient will eventually be diagnosed with diabetes. And while all this is going on, the only symptom that is usually present is that of low energy.

Stress as a Major Factor Increasing the Complications of Diabetes

I just described how chronic stress can often play an important role in the genesis of diabetes, but an even more critical aspect of stress is how it can dramatically worsen not only diabetes itself but also most of the complications of diabetes. For example, because excessive cortisol causes an increase in blood sugar levels, stress often makes it quite difficult for someone with diabetes to achieve optimum glucose control.

Chronic stress also triggers and intensifies many of the complications of diabetes, such as the following:

- Increased blood pressure

- Increased cholesterol levels

- Atherosclerosis

- Insomnia

- Interference with deep-stage sleep

- Decreased immune response

With a list like this, it's no wonder that virtually all healthcare professionals agree that decreasing the stress response is critical to maintaining optimum heath. It certainly is crucial for preventing and treating type 2 diabetes. And the good news is that decreasing your stress response is a lot easier than you might imagine.

WHERE DOES STRESS COME FROM?

Let's get one thing clear from the start. Stress doesn't come from "out there." We make it all ourselves, 100 percent of it. When my wife is "stressing me out," it's really me stressing myself out over what she is doing or saying. When I look at the condition of the world, and it is "stressing me out," it's really a case of me stressing myself out over the condition of the world. This is both the good and bad news.

The bad news first: you, not someone or something else, are creating *all* of your stress. If you need to blame someone for your stress level, blame yourself. This fact leads to the really good news: since you are creating all of your stress, then it is within your power to get rid of it. If this were not the case, if your stresses were in fact caused by forces outside of yourself, the whole thing would be fairly hopeless, since you would then have to control or direct what is going on outside of yourself in order to remove the source of the stress.

The false belief that stress is caused by external factors, which on one level or another we have all come to accept, is behind the epidemic of stress that we now have in the modern world. When you believe that stress is caused by factors outside of yourself, there are only two responses you can have, a feeling of hopelessness or a desire to control your environment, both of which I see all day long in my clinic.

The first response is hopelessness. This is a very natural response—if you believe that stress is caused by external factors, and you are savvy enough to realize that you cannot control these factors, then in fact you are right, the situation is quite hopeless. I see hopelessness in the faces of many of my diabetic patients because they have been falsely led to believe that diabetes and the consequences of diabetes are beyond their control. This is the biggest single reason why those with diabetes fail to stick to their programs even when they are working. When we are feeling hopeless about things, we often fall into sabotaging behaviors like craving donuts because "what's the use anyway?" On the other hand, when we realize that all our stress, including the stresses associated with having diabetes, is caused by ourselves, then we will realize that it is well within our power to eliminate it, and hopelessness will fly away.

The second response to the belief that stress is caused by outside factors is to control your environment. In my case, this means making my wife wrong and/or telling her to change her ways simply because what she is saying or doing is making me feel uncomfortable. It means getting upset with your boss and trying to change him because he doesn't have a clue, and isn't able to see what needs to be done even when you tell him. It often means avoiding situations and people, even friends, because they just can't see the light in the same way that you do and won't change to be more like you. In its unfriendliest terms, this stress response involves manipulating our environment so that it is the way we want it to be.

This response to stress is what also causes us to be obsessive in our concern over the future, doing everything we can to make sure that absolutely nothing will go wrong. So obsessed are we by what is likely to happen tomorrow that we are often not present for today. When my computer blinks out, I go crazy because I have taken all the necessary precautions, in other words, "it wasn't supposed to happen." This control response to stress is very common. People with diabetes who fall into this pattern often get so stressed out over the details of their treatment that the whole process becomes overwhelming, and they become forced to find a way or an excuse to get off their program.

RESPONDING TO STRESS

The way to avoid both of these pitfalls, that is, hopelessness and a compulsive need to control your environment, is to recognize that 100 percent of your stress is caused by you. That's right, 100 percent. Once you get that idea into your head, you are going in the right direction, because all of us have the power to change ourselves, and none of us have the power to change very much outside of ourselves.

So how do we manage to create all this stress for ourselves? The full answer to this question is certainly well beyond the scope of this book, but I will give you some very good ideas that I have learned from all of the wonderful patients I have had over the years.

I believe that the major reason for stress is what the psychologists call "attachment." Attachment refers to the difference between wanting something and believing that we need it. When we believe that we need something, we are "attached" to it. For example, I want to be loved. That's just a simple want or desire. However, if I start to believe that I *need* to be loved in order to be happy or secure, then I become attached to the idea of being loved.

In this way, attachment is a sure recipe for stress because we end up betting all of our happiness on whether or not we obtain something that ultimately is beyond our control, and that therefore we may not get. The cure for avoiding the pitfalls of attachment is to stop needing and just stick with wanting. Your stress will evaporate to the extent that you are willing to do this.

Attachment is a lose-lose situation. There's no way we can win. Here's what happens when we attach to something: either we get that thing—for example, I manage to find someone who really loves me—or I don't. If, in the first scenario, I do find someone who loves me, then my stress results from the fact that I have finally found the thing that I need so badly, and I start to become stressed over the possibility of losing it. I might become jealous. I might become easily offended at any remark other than "I love you, you're the best." God only knows what lengths I will go to in order to make sure that that person loves me, because I *need* the love. The likelihood, in fact, is pretty good that this need of mine may cause me to behave in a way that ironically leads to the person no longer loving me.

The problem with the second possible outcome stemming from attachment is more obvious. If I don't get the thing I think I need in order to be happy, content, or secure, then I can't be happy, content, or secure, and I will be stressed over that. Either way, once you attach yourself to something, whether it's a person, a job, or just an idea or concept, you are automatically on the highway to stress.

Oh, by the way, the same problems emerge if instead of attaching yourself to the idea that you need something, you attach yourself to the idea that you need to get rid of something. Examples abound: "I need to get rid of my debts to be happy," "I need to get rid of my husband to be happy," and so forth.

One of my favorite attachments is the need to have everything go right. I don't know where or when I decided that I needed this, but somewhere along the line, I bought it hook, line, and sinker. So when something doesn't go quite as I want (did I say need?) it to, and I become stressed as a result, I can quickly eliminate the stress by just realizing that though I may have wanted things to turn out differently, I don't need them to be different in order to be happy.

So just remember this the next time you are feeling stressed over something. Behind your stress is probably the belief that you need some thing in order to be happy, content, or secure. Your job is to figure out what it is you believe you need so much that you can't be happy without it. Once you examine that belief, you may very well find that although you want it, you really don't need it. That's when your stress level will very quickly dissipate, and you will have done a lot to improve both your glucose control and the overall quality of your life. In fact, when you really think about it, there are only four things you actually need: food, water, shelter, and air—the rest are just wants.

BREATHING AIR IN—BREATHING STRESS OUT

The New Zealand short-story writer Katherine Mansfield once wrote, "By health I mean the power to live a full, adult, living, breathing life in close contact with the earth and the wonders thereof—the sea—the sun." Breathing is elemental—like eating. You do it or else. An absolutely amazing way to soften the effects of stress on your physiology is by working with your breathing.

Modern science has given us all the physiological details about what occurs in the breathing process, but ancient thinkers had already focused attention on this issue long before we had such detailed understanding. The ancients quite naturally reasoned that since *not* breathing was synonymous with death, breathing itself must be pretty important, and that there must be both proper and improper ways to breathe.

It turns out that they were quite right. There is a right and a wrong way to breathe. And all too frequently, we do it the wrong way. Improper breathing is, in fact, a major—and widely ignored—cause of stress, panic attacks, anxiety, low energy, and premature aging. This became very clear to me soon after I began using Bio-Energy Testing, which revealed that improper breathing resulted in a fairly significant decrease in energy production caused by insufficient oxygen delivery at the capillary level.

There are two really quite different ways to breathe: one is known as *chest-wall breathing* and the other is called *diaphragmatic* or *abdominal breathing*. Chest-wall breathing employs the chest, shoulder, and neck muscles to lift up the chest in order to inflate the lungs. As you inhale, the chest expands and the abdomen is sucked in. This is the classic "chest out, abdomen in" form of breathing taught in the military and reinforced in our culture all throughout youth. To determine if you are a "chest breather," just sit quietly in a chair, resting and breathing easily, and observe how your chest and abdomen move when you inhale. If your abdomen does not go out every time you inhale, and/or if your chest expands, you are chest breathing. This is not the preferred "style." As we will discuss in a moment, there are several reasons why this type of breathing aggravates and even causes chronic anxiety.

In diaphragmatic or abdominal breathing, on the other hand, your abdomen bulges out when you inhale and your chest remains still. This means you are using the diaphragm, an internal muscle located at the bottom of the chest cage, to draw in the air. As the diaphragm expands downward, the abdomen naturally expands along with it. This is the preferred "style."

The Shortcomings of Chest-Wall Breathing

Chest-wall breathing fails to draw as much oxygen into the lung's air sacs as does abdominal breathing. Here's why: The lungs have what is known in pulmonary physiology as "dead space." This refers simply to the space taken up by the tubes (airways) through which the air passes en route to the air sacs, where oxygen is delivered to the bloodstream. The airways are thus "dead space" in that they don't participate in the actual oxygen exchange. It turns out that the upper part of the lungs has more dead space than the lower part.

Chest-wall breathing selectively fills the upper part of the lungs, whereas abdominal breathing selectively fills the lower part. Thus, the former is less efficient in the mechanics of oxygen acquisition.

In order to make up for the decreased amount of oxygen acquired per breath, chest-wall breathers automatically compensate by increasing their respiratory rate, often as high as twelve to eighteen breaths per minute. By comparison, an abdominal breather usually needs only six to eight breaths per minute to acquire the same volume of oxygen.

Chest-wall breathers are obviously working harder to acquire the same amount of oxygen as an abdominal breather. That's only part of the problem. The increased respiratory rate associated with chest-wall breathing is known as "chronic sub-acute hyperventilation." It can be clearly detected by Bio-Energy Testing because it results in an excessive excretion of carbon dioxide. The increased loss of carbon dioxide shifts the pH of the blood in the brain and in the rest of the body into a state known as alkalosis, often leading to chronic, unexplained anxiety. Alkalosis also results in decreased oxygen delivery to every cell in the body. Let me explain how.

When you breathe in oxygen, it gets taken up by the hemoglobin molecule contained in your red blood cells. Hemoglobin has an incredibly strong attraction for oxygen. It holds tightly to the oxygen as it passes though the arterial network and down to the level of the cells, where oxygen is delivered. As we have already seen, the hemoglobin molecule releases its oxygen cargo in the presence of the enzyme 2,3 DPG, which is often deficient in those with diabetes.

But the hemoglobin molecule is also triggered into releasing oxygen in response to the acid it encounters at the cellular level. A problem can then occur if the normal acid balance becomes disrupted due to the alkalosis caused by chest-wall breathing. This effectively prevents the hemoglobin molecule from releasing its oxygen. The result is a decrease in available oxygen to the cells and a decrease in energy production.

If you have ever gone through a very stressful period—and who hasn't—you may have noticed that afterward you feel drained and fatigued. One reason for this is that stress almost always puts people into a chest-wall-breathing mode. And, as you've just read, this contributes to low energy through the alkalosis effect.

Emergency Response

Since respiration is designed to operate more efficiently through abdominal breathing, you might be wondering why our bodies developed the ability to chest-wall breathe. The answer has to do with how and when the brain senses peril.

In emergency situations, the body requires additional oxygen. In the distant past, you would have needed a major injection of oxygen to flee from a lion that had targeted you for its next meal. To meet such threatening challenges, the body kicks into a double-breathing mode—chest-wall combined with abdominal breathing. This quickly sucks in an extra supply of oxygen.

In intense situations like these, where exertion is at an ultra-peak level, alkalosis does not occur. Oxygen uptake and delivery are maximized. Thus, the body evolved the capability of chest breathing as a survival mechanism.

Although survival and escape from life-threatening predicaments may not be part of daily existence for most of us, the everyday variety of mental anguish and stresses experienced in modern living is enough to switch on the chest-wall-breathing response. The unconscious part of the brain reads this initiation of chest-wall breathing as a sign of an impending danger, and triggers anxiety attacks.

You may just be sitting in your car worrying about running late for an appointment. Unbeknownst to you, the tension causes you to begin to chest-wall breathe, and then *whamo*, your brain senses danger and suddenly goes into an emergency mode. You may then experience a panicky feeling, which is all the more stressful because there is no apparent reason why you should have such a reaction.

A Vicious Cycle

Chronic chest-wall breathing generates a vicious cycle. As discussed, it causes the following conditions:

- Increased respiration

- Alkalosis, resulting in decreased oxygen consumption

- Decreased energy production

- An emergency mode in the body

- Anxiety and stress

All of this promotes even more chest-wall breathing. And if you throw in a stressful event, you can readily see how an anxiety attack can develop. When anxiety becomes chronic, most people will run to the doctor and get a prescription for a sedative. The medication slows down the respiratory rate and seems to correct the problem. However, the sedative only takes care of the symptoms, and does not correct the root problem. Often, it creates new problems in terms of side effects.

A healthier way is to teach yourself to breathe with your diaphragm. The alternative is to continue the habit of chest-wall breathing, which will deprive you of optimal energy and cause you to age faster.

How to Breathe the Right Way

Diaphragmatic breathing is one of the very first techniques that singers and musicians are taught in order to provide them with ample air for those long notes. I personally learned the method years ago in a yoga class, and it gave me a significant advantage later when I was actively involved in competitive cycling.

The technique is quite simple, but you may need some guidance because it is somewhat subtle. Once you've got the idea, it just takes a little practice over a few months to fully perfect it and make it automatic. When I was learning the technique, I made up little signs saying "breathe!" I put them everywhere: on my watch, my dashboard, my bike, my mirror. The signs were reminders to check how I was breathing. And when I checked, I was usually breathing with my chest. In that case I would just take a few good abdominal breaths and try to concentrate on breathing this way as much as possible. I also spent a few minutes every morning and evening performing breath meditation.

I will explain breath meditation in a moment, but first follow these few simple steps to learn the diaphragmatic technique. Most people can grasp the basic movement within a few minutes. Here's what to do:

1. Lie down on your back. It's hard to chest-wall breathe while lying down. Even the most "die-hard" chest breathers tend to breathe with the diaphragm in this position.

2. Now place your hand on your abdomen and notice how it rises slightly when you inhale and goes down when you exhale. This movement is the hallmark of breathing with your diaphragm. If you are breathing with your chest, your hand will not elevate during the inhale, but will instead drop down. If you are naturally breathing with your diaphragm

while lying down, you are well on your way. If it isn't coming naturally, don't worry. Just give it a bit more time. You'll get it soon enough.

3. After you finally become familiar with the feel of diaphragmatic breathing, I would like you to practice an exaggerated form by contracting your abdominal muscles inward (sucking in your gut) as you exhale the air from your lungs. Then expand the same muscles outward to inhale. Keep practicing this technique until you can breathe fully and somewhat deeply without moving your chest. If the movement doesn't come easily, enroll the help of a spouse or friend or yoga instructor to help you.

4. Once you have learned this exaggerated form lying down, try the same thing while sitting in a chair, and then while standing. Finally, to perfect your newly discovered "talent," try doing it while you are singing in the shower or exercising. You can then proudly announce to friends and family that you have at last learned to breathe correctly!

There are additional benefits to diaphragmatic breathing that should help inspire you. One is that it often helps to eliminate or significantly reduce neck pain and tension commonly caused by chronically raising up the chest during chest-wall breathing. Diaphragmatic breathing does not create any neck and shoulder strain since it moves with gravity instead of against it. It also strengthens and tightens the abdominal muscles. And finally, it often benefits individuals with asthma or other lung conditions.

Using Breath Meditation to Soften the Effects of Stress

Perhaps nothing is as powerful as the mind to either make us sick or keep us healthy. But how can we learn to harness and direct that power? One tried-and-true method is breath meditation.

This meditative exercise is particularly effective against stress-related disorders, insomnia, and hypertension. It also generates more energy and stamina. In addition, it's a very effective way to train your mind to work better for you. That means increased mental clarity, speed, and memory. Moreover, breath meditation is completely free and devoid of side effects. No gyms to join or pills to take! The little time it takes to do it will very typically lead to many wonderful rewards.

To start with, let's get the concept straight. Meditation, at least the way I'm using the word, refers to mental exercise. Meditation and prayer are not the same thing. Praying is a different concept. It has its own powers, but is *not* a substitute for meditation. So even if you regularly pray, please be sure to practice some form of meditation, as well.

Breath meditation trains the conscious mind to focus better and the unconscious mind to relax better. It works in the same way that training your muscles makes them function better.

Often, you will find your meditation session to be relaxing. But there will also be many days in which emotions or stresses may preoccupy your mind and you may find yourself expending more effort to meditate. Don't worry about that. It's normal. If that did not happen then there would be no real reason for you to meditate in the first place. Just take it as it comes and apply the simple guidelines given in this chapter. What's important to understand here is that no matter how relaxing a meditation session may or may not be, it will still serve to improve your overall relaxation potential and strengthen your powers of concentration.

Your Mind Is Like a Puppy

Your mind is like a puppy. It wants to wander around and experience everything it can. This is a wonderful thing, but it can also limit the mind's ability to focus, and mental power is directly related to focus. Breath meditation trains your mind to better focus, and in so doing strengthens your mental power. This increases the ease with which you do everything!

The process takes fifteen to twenty minutes. If you can do it regularly once or twice a day, it may be the most productive fifteen or twenty minutes of "doing nothing" that you can possibly imagine. Just follow the easy steps and you'll be on your way.

Step 1: The Setting

First, ideally you should have some quiet space, a room where you can meditate without interruption. If there's a phone in the room, pull out the plug. You'll also need a comfortable chair, one with armrests if possible. Sit comfortably. Don't cross your legs. Take three deep relaxing breaths, and when you exhale the third time, let your eyes close.

Step 2: Control Breathing

Use the diaphragmatic breathing technique you just learned. Now you're going to "control breathe." By that I mean, pause to hold your breath at the end of both your inhale and your exhale. The pauses should be the same length of time that you use to breathe. For example, if you inhale (expanding your abdomen in the process) over a two-second period, then hold your breath for a two-second pause before you begin to exhale. Then exhale (sucking in your abdomen) over a two-second interval. At the end of your exhale, pause for two seconds before you begin the next breath. If you inhale over a three-second count, then just make sure that the other intervals are three-seconds long. Keep repeating this process for each and every breath. It's as simple as that!

You can count the seconds to yourself as you go along, but after a while you will probably find that you are able to naturally keep the intervals the same without counting. Just remember to breathe only with your abdomen. Keep your chest free of movement.

While you go through this routine, there are several things to be aware of, including sighs and yawns and the need to alter your breathing rate.

Sighs and yawns. Most people experience the need to sigh about every ten minutes. During meditation, when you feel the urge to sigh, just go with it. Remember that sighing invokes both chest-wall and diaphragmatic breathing. After the sigh, simply return to controlled abdominal breathing. Sometimes you may feel the urge to sigh but it just doesn't develop. This just means that your body doesn't need one yet. Sighs are relaxing, but don't force them. Be patient. One will come along soon enough.

Don't be bothered by yawning. I can remember many times when I have yawned as many as twenty times during a meditation session. Just go with it, and as soon as the yawn passes, simply return to controlled abdominal breathing.

Altering your breathing rate. One thing sure to happen while you are practicing breath meditation is that you will need to alter your breathing rate to accommodate how you feel. If you feel breathless or have "air hunger," you will need to increase the rate. This is often noticed during the pause at the end of an exhalation.

When you notice this, simply increase your breathing rate so that you are comfortable and no longer feel in need of air. For example, if you are breathing in two-second intervals and you feel breathless, decrease the intervals to one second. This adjustment will cause your breathing rate to increase and get rid of the breathless feeling.

Conversely, as the session progresses and your body becomes more relaxed, you will usually need to *decrease* your breathing rate. If you start to feel a little dizzy as if you are hyperventilating or breathing too fast, just decrease your breathing rate accordingly by *increasing* the length of the intervals. You may very likely have to adjust your breathing rate a few times during a session in order to maintain comfort.

Step 3: Training the Puppy

A crucial part of breath meditation is your mental focus. While you are sitting there comfortably using your abdominal muscles to practice controlled breathing, it is important that you keep your mind entirely focused on your breathing. You can focus on your breathing rate, how the air feels in your lungs, or how your abdomen feels as it moves in and out. It doesn't matter exactly what you focus on, as long as it has something to do with your breathing.

But remember what I said a moment ago about the mind being like a very inquisitive and active puppy. It may not always reconcile itself with the drill called meditation. Imagine having a puppy on a leash and training it to sit comfortably by your side. As soon as you place the puppy on the floor next to you, it will immediately begin to wander in one direction or another. Without becoming upset with the puppy, just imagine yourself gently retrieving it, and putting it next to you again.

Your mind is going to stray the same way. No matter how hard you try to keep your attention on your breathing, the mind will wander off into this thought or that thought. Just like with the puppy, as soon as you become aware that your mind is wandering, gently retrieve it, and refocus on your breathing.

This repetitive cycle of concentrating, straying, and refocusing is the nature of breath meditation. The more you practice this retrieving and refocusing, the stronger your power of concentration will be. After several months of regular practice, you will begin to notice that the mind is wandering less, and that you are retrieving your awareness more easily. Although your mind is an extremely stubborn puppy, it will eventually learn.

People who continue meditating in this fashion greatly limit the negative effects of stress on their physiology. They see an improvement in virtually every health function measured. The practice contributes to longer and healthier life. Don't underestimate the power of this simple exercise to increase your energy levels, enhance your mental speed and concentration, and improve your mood, sleep, and emotional state.

WHAT ELSE?

I don't want to end this chapter without mentioning two books that I believe encapsulate everything any of us needs to know about stress. The first book is by a remarkable woman by the name of Byron Katie (no I didn't write her name backwards). Ms. Katie has written an extraordinary book by the name of *Loving What Is.* For those of you who would like to get a better handle on how to discover and deal with those attachments that are causing you stress, I don't know of a better book. In fact, I would rather have you listen to her CD recording of the book than read the book, but many of my patients have found great value in doing both. Her book and CD by the same name can be purchased at www.thework.org.

The other reference I want to give you is a book called *The Power of the Now* by Eckhart Tolle. Mr. Tolle does an unbelievably good job of explaining how essentially all of our stress is a result of putting our conscious attention on either the past or the future instead of the present moment. This simple concept is one that probably all of us have contemplated at some time or another, but, like most simple concepts, just gets ignored. To put it another way, to the degree that we can focus our attention on what is happening in the present moment, we will be able to virtually eliminate all stress. Eckhart Tolle's book describes why this is so, and also offers some very effective techniques for staying in the present moment or, as he calls it, the now. Once again, I will advise you to get not only the book but especially the recorded CD. They can be purchased at any bookstore.

The reason I always recommend the recorded CDs in addition to these books is that you can play the CDs over and over again as you drive in your car, walk, or ride the bus. The bad habits that we all have that cause our stress are so thoroughly ingrained in our being that it often takes listening to these corrective ideas again and again over an extended period of time.

CHAPTER 12

STEP SEVEN:
Correcting Hormone Imbalances

They always say time changes things,
but actually you have to change them yourself.
—ANDY WARHOL, ARTIST (1928–1987)

Ignoring the overriding importance of hormones is one of the major mistakes commonly made in the conventional treatment and prevention of diabetes. Although much emphasis is placed on the hormone insulin, the other important hormones—the thyroid hormones, testosterone, cortisol, DHEA, and growth hormone—are usually ignored. I have found over and over again that the proper replacement of hormones as they become deficient is absolutely essential to the successful prevention and management of diabetes. In this chapter I will explain how maintaining an appropriate hormone balance acts to improve energy production, increase fat metabolism, and decrease insulin resistance. Additionally, please note that it is not just hormonal deficiencies that can be a problem. In the case of cortisol and growth hormone, an excess can literally cause diabetes as well as decrease blood sugar control.

WHAT ARE HORMONES ANYWAY?

Hormones are the messengers that run the body. They orchestrate your digestion. They organize and regulate your immune system response. They affect the way you think and even your mood. There is no function in the human body that is not significantly impacted by your hormones. But perhaps the most important function of hormones is that they control and adjust virtually every aspect of your metabolism and energy production. If you agree with me that a deficit of energy is the root cause of aging and disease, you can then begin to appreciate how incredibly important your hormones are not only to the quality of your life but also to your longevity.

There are hormones that make your body selectively burn fat for energy, and there are opposing hormones that act to shunt your body into burning glucose for energy. There are hormones that increase your energy production, and conversely, hormones that act to reduce energy production.

For every hormone that does one thing, there is usually another hormone that does the opposite. This is how your body regulates itself according to its needs. Thus, you can see that it is not just the absolute amount of any one hormone that is significant, but more importantly, it is the balance between all the hormones.

IS NATURAL HORMONE REPLACEMENT SAFE?

Many people don't have a good understanding of just exactly what is meant by natural hormone replacement. If they did, I would not hear the question over and over again from my patients, "But is it healthy for me?"

Just stop and think about it. If you will agree with me that young adults aged thirty to forty are generally the healthiest people in the population, then you must also agree that this age bracket must have the healthiest balance of hormones, since hormones are so crucial to health. All natural hormonal replacement means is that we are working to reestablish the healthy balance of hormones that you had when you were young but lost as you grew older. By so doing we are able to do an awful lot to keep your fat and oxygen metabolism very close to those of a young person, thus drastically slowing down the processes involved in aging and in the development of diseases such as diabetes.

WHERE DID MY HORMONES GO?

But let me make a little digression here and ask another question. Since hormones are so valuable to our health and overall physical function, why is it that Mother Nature causes hormone levels to go down as we get older?

Well, the warm and fuzzy answer to that question is pretty obvious when you stop to consider it. By the age of forty, you probably will have already mated, added to the gene pool, and propagated the race, and from a preservation-of-the-species perspective, Mother Nature no longer has a need for you. You have in a sense outlived your usefulness.

Okay, so that's the common-sense version, but is there a more scientific explanation? The scientific answer was first formulated in the early

1950s by Vladimir Dilman, Ph.D., who postulated what he called the neuroendocrine theory of aging.

Dilman noted that when we are first born we are immediately thrust into a period of rapid growth and development, and that this period lasts for about eighteen to twenty years before it slows down and eventually stops. Dilman reasoned that if Nature had not evolved a way to curtail the rapid growth and development we experience as children and adolescents, we would continue to grow and would ultimately die prematurely as a consequence of excessive growth.

He knew that it was hormones that regulated the rate of growth and development, and that it was the nervous system that regulated the release of those hormones. Therefore, he proposed the following theory: the control mechanisms in the brain that regulate hormone release start to turn off the flow of hormones in the late teenage years, and this decline in hormone production just continues to plummet as we get older.

As a matter of a fact, a steady and predictable decline is exactly what is seen when hormone levels are measured in persons as they become older. Of course, as these hormone levels decline, so does energy production. Eventually the levels become so low that, combined with other factors, such as stress, sleep deficiency, dietary carbohydrate, and nutritional deficiencies, an energy deficit results.

HORMONE REPLACEMENT:
THE RIGHT WAY AND THE WRONG WAY

Natural hormone replacement simply refers to the process of measuring exactly how low the levels of a given hormone have become, and correcting the deficiency by adding in the missing amount using either a pill or an injection. Sounds easy, doesn't it? It is, but unfortunately not all physicians do this in concert with the way that Nature works. There are three mistakes that I commonly see being made by physicians not trained in natural hormone replacement.

First, they often don't replace the declining hormone with the identical hormone. For example, physicians frequently use a synthetic version of testosterone called methyltestosterone to replace natural testosterone. Another example is when physicians use the drug Provera to replace the natural hormone progesterone. As my friend and pioneer in the science of natural hormone replacement Jonathan Wright, M.D., often states, "This is like using airplane parts to replace automobile parts." It's not a good idea, and often leads to side effects combined with decreased efficacy.

Second, many physicians don't seem to realize that due to the incredible diversity of human physiology, a dosage that is perfect for one person may be completely inappropriate for someone else. Here is a dramatic example of the variability that can be seen among individuals: one in twenty women well into her menopausal years still manufactures a significant amount of estrogen. Who would have guessed that the estrogen levels of a menopausal woman are adequate, and that she doesn't need any replacement at all? Of course, other women will require anywhere from a slightly higher dose to a significantly higher dose, compared to average, depending on how their particular bodies work.

When I am prescribing natural hormones for my patients, I always make certain to follow not only their clinical responses (that is, their physical signs and symptoms) but also the laboratory levels of the hormones I am replacing. In this way, after a series of trying various doses and comparing the clinical and laboratory results, it is possible to determine exactly how much of the hormone an individual patient's body requires. The correct prescription is then custom manufactured for that person by a compounding pharmacist. In this way, I am able to avoid all of the problems associated with the one-size-fits-all mentality.

The third mistake that is commonly seen occurs when a physician forgets the important interplay that occurs between hormones, and only replaces the one he or she is concerned with. For example, a man sees his physician for symptoms associated with testosterone deficiency, and the physician replaces his testosterone without also paying attention to his levels of growth hormone, thyroid, or estradiol.

All hormones affect one another, and this interplay is variable from individual to individual. Without closely monitoring and treating *all* of a patient's hormones, a physician may be playing Russian roulette by simply replacing the one he or she is clinically interested in. In my opinion, it is really nothing more than common sense to replace hormones in such a way as to maintain the same balance that Nature has already established.

When it comes to diabetes, proper natural replacement of insulin, thyroid hormones, cortisol, DHEA, testosterone, and growth hormone is absolutely essential for optimal success. And for those all those millions of people out there who don't have diabetes yet but are on the road to the disease, the natural replacement of deficient hormones is often critical to preventing the disease.

CORRECTING INSULIN IMBALANCE

Of course, when discussing diabetes the very first hormone that comes to mind is insulin. It is insulin that allows glucose to get into the cells.

You will remember that diabetes develops from a condition I call pre-diabetes, in which the cells of the body become insensitive or resistant to the effects of insulin. In this stage there is no elevation of blood sugar because the pancreas is able to counteract the cells' resistance to insulin by simply making more of the hormone. Ultimately, however, the islet cells of the pancreas, which make insulin, will become worn out by this excessive activity, and the insulin levels will begin to decrease. It is at this point that diabetes can be diagnosed by an elevation in the blood glucose levels.

If diabetes is diagnosed at a time when the pancreas still has enough islet cells left to make insulin, the conventional treatment at this point is to prescribe one or more of three classes of medications. One class of medications can be referred to as insulin sensitizers. These drugs work by helping the body use insulin more efficiently, resulting both in better blood sugar control and in lower levels of insulin. Commonly used drugs in this class are metformin (Glucophage), rosiglitazone (Avandia), and pioglitazone (Actos). Although I only need to prescribe medications to those patients who either won't follow the program or who were beyond rescue when I first met them, insulin sensitizers are my favorites for several reasons:

- They just plain make sense since diabetes always comes with insulin resistance.

- They do not appear to cause weight gain.

- They improve cholesterol readings.

- They are much less likely to trigger low blood sugar than the sulfonylureas discussed below.

Another class of drugs for type 2 diabetes includes acarbose (Precose) and miglitol (Glyset). These medications work by delaying the digestion of sugar and starch, thereby leveling off the spikes in blood sugar that follow meals. I don't really like these drugs, mostly because my patients don't eat carbohydrate in the first place, so they wouldn't need to take a drug to interfere with carbohydrate absorption. Also, since these drugs interfere with digestion, they have a lot of aggravating side effects such as gas, diarrhea, and cramping.

The third class of medications is made up of the sulfonylureas. These include tolbutamide (Orinase), chlorpropamide (Diabinese), tolazamide (Tolinase), glyburide (Micronase, Glynase, DiaBeta), glimepiride (Amaryl), and glipizide (Glucotrol). Sulfonylureas work by stimulating the pancreas to make more insulin. These are my least favorite drugs because stimulating the pancreas in a diabetic is like beating a tired horse.

Although sulfonylureas can be very helpful in controlling blood sugars, they should only be used as a last resort. By forcing an already overburdened pancreas to produce more insulin, they will hasten the ultimate destruction of the pancreatic islet cells from excessive free-radical damage. If and when all of the islet cells of the pancreas become destroyed, the pancreas will be unable to manufacture any insulin at all. This state of insulin deficiency is the most advanced state of diabetes, and is referred to as insulin-dependent diabetes. When a patient reaches this stage, he or she will require daily insulin injections for the remainder of his or her life.

One of the goals of writing this book is to educate you on all the various forms of therapy you can use to control your diabetes without having to resort to the use of pancreas-stimulating drugs like the sulfonylureas. In this way, it is possible to insure that you will never become insulin dependent.

Insulin Replacement Therapy

My job as a primary care physician has not been focused on the final stage of insulin dependency, but rather on preventing my patients from ever getting to that point. To that end, if you are diagnosed with diabetes at a time when your pancreas is still able to make insulin, and you follow the recommendations in this book, it is highly unlikely that you will ever require insulin replacement therapy.

However, if you have already been advised by your doctor that your pancreas no longer makes insulin, you have no choice but to replace your deficient hormone levels with regular insulin injections. In this case, let me refer you to an excellent book written by Richard Bernstein, M.D., entitled *Dr. Bernstein's Diabetes Solution*. Dr. Bernstein does an absolutely fabulous job at explaining the ins and outs of insulin replacement therapy. It is very important to note, though, that it is still highly beneficial for you to follow the recommendations in this book, because doing so will result in both a decreased need for insulin, and a decrease in the complications that often occur with insulin replacement.

Testing for Insulin Deficiency or Excess

There are two really good ways to test insulin levels. One is simply to obtain a fasting blood level around eight in the morning. The patient should not exercise before the blood is taken. As I've mentioned before, although the standard reference range shows "normal" values to be between 5 and 25 microunits per milliliter (mU/ml), this simply reflects the elevated insulin levels that we "normally" have in this country as a result of the typical American lifestyle and eating habits. In actuality, perfect insulin levels are below 7 mU/ml. Any level over 10 mU/ml is too high and should be treated.

But just checking out insulin levels can be very misleading because many patients have elevated levels only after eating and/or are able to clear the elevated insulin levels very quickly. So, just to be sure, if I have a patient with diabetes who has an insulin level below 10 mU/ml, I will then get a blood C-peptide level. C-peptide is a molecule that is formed in the body as a result of insulin production, and therefore serves as a good indicator of how much insulin the body is producing. It is often a better way of assessing insulin output because it remains more constant in the blood and cannot be cleared as quickly as insulin can be.

CORRECTING THYROID HORMONE IMBALANCE

As we know, diabetes is an energy deficit disorder. It is caused in genetically sensitive individuals by an overall decrease in energy production combined with a shift from fat metabolism to glucose metabolism. Because thyroid hormones are intimately involved in both of these areas, adequate levels of these hormones are absolutely crucial to the optimum control and prevention of diabetes. Let's look at the effect of thyroid hormones on energy production.

Thyroid Hormones and Energy Production

The thyroid gland, in conjunction with a properly functioning liver, produces two hormones, T3 and T4. It turns out that energy production rates are drastically affected by the levels of these hormones. According to Arthur C. Guyton's classic *Textbook of Medical Physiology*, "Both of these hormones have the profound effect of increasing the metabolic rate of the body." Guyton goes on to point out that over 50 percent of the entire energy capacity of the body is fully dependent on thyroid hormones alone!

This is truly a remarkable observation when one considers that a deficiency of either of these hormones is quite common in the general population and even more common in those with diabetes. It's also no wonder that the symptoms associated with a deficiency of thyroid hormones, a condition referred to as hypothyroidism, reads like a litany of what can go wrong in the human body.

More than half of American men and women over the age of forty experience *three or more* symptoms related to hypothyroidism. And over the age of fifty, I find that it is fairly uncommon to have optimal levels of thyroid hormones. Common symptoms and signs of thyroid hormone deficiency are as follows:

- Fatigue
- Decreased stamina and endurance
- Elevated cholesterol
- Low body temperature
- Acne
- Dry, scaly, coarse, pale-looking skin
- Puffy, water-retentive skin that is cool to the touch
- Vitamin B_{12} deficiency
- Heartburn
- Failure to digest food adequately
- Low resting heart rate (normally 60–70 beats per minute)

- Low blood pressure
- Weak pulse
- Enlarged tongue
- Dry, brittle, lackluster hair
- Loss of hair on eyebrows and legs
- Weak fingernails
- Vitamin A deficiency (thyroid converts carotene to vitamin A)
- Weight gain
- Slow wound healing
- Frequent cold and flu viruses
- Heat intolerance
- Cold intolerance

- Decreased appetite
- Diminished libido, impotence, anorgasmia
- Menstrual disturbances
- Premenstrual syndrome (PMS)
- Chronic dry eyes
- Constipation
- Joint pain
- Headaches (especially migraines)
- Raynaud's phenomenon
- Carpal tunnel syndrome

Those with diabetes and their physicians often assume that many of the above-listed symptoms are just part of diabetes, but in truth, they are often caused by undiagnosed hypothyroidism. As you will see below, the diagnosis of this disease is very commonly missed in conventional medicine.

Thyroid Hormones and Fat Metabolism

Besides energy production in general, thyroid hormones are also critical for the metabolism of fat, and when they are deficient, the body is forced to rely more and more on glucose metabolism. Again to quote Guyton, "Essentially all aspects of fat metabolism are enhanced under the influence of thyroid hormones." That's a powerful statement and one that I have found to be very true in my clinical practice. In fact, the very first step of fat metabolism, in which the stored fat in adipose tissue is broken down to be used by the cells, is completely dependent on the presence of thyroid hormones.

The effect of a deficiency of thyroid hormones on fat metabolism is also exemplified by elevated blood fats such as cholesterol, particularly the "bad cholesterol" called LDL (low-density lipoprotein) cholesterol. Many patients and physicians alike are often unaware of the significance of the relationship between thyroid hormone deficiency and high cholesterol: hypothyroidism was originally diagnosed, in the first half of the twentieth century, by elevated cholesterol levels.

The primary reason that as people get older their cholesterol goes up stems from decreased thyroid hormone production. Elevated cholesterol is a benchmark indicator of low thyroid function.

Thyroid Hormones Are the Master Hormones

Of all the hormones in the body, the thyroid hormones are referred to as the "master hormones." There are two reasons for this.

First of all, since hormones are produced in glands as a consequence of energy production, when thyroid hormones are deficient, these hormone-producing glands just can't synthesize their hormones as well as they need to. This is why patients with hypothyroidism often show a deficiency in many other hormones as a result.

And, yes, low levels of thyroid hormones also result in a decreased production of insulin. Ironically enough, since thyroid hormones are produced in the thyroid gland, low thyroid-hormone levels even cause a decreased production of themselves! As a result of this latter observation, I often find that the correct dose of thyroid hormone that is needed to adequately replace a patient's deficiency will often have to be lowered later on, as his or her thyroid gland responds to the treatment and starts to produce more hormones on its own.

Secondly, the thyroid hormones exert what is described in the physiology texts as a "permissive effect" on many other hormones. What this means is that in order for other hormones to exert their particular activity, the thyroid hormones need to be present. Thus, in a state of thyroid hormone deficiency, even though other hormones such as growth hormone and cortisol may be present in adequate amounts, they will not be able to function adequately. The end result will be the same as if they were deficient.

Between the control over hormone synthesis and the permissive effect, you can see why thyroid hormones are so important for optimal functioning of all the hormones. They are, indeed, the master hormones.

Diagnosing Hypothyroidism

You would think that diagnosing hypothyroidism would be pretty easy given how common it is, but unfortunately this is not the case precisely because it is so common. Many patients with hypothyroidism go undiagnosed and are forever relegated to various levels of permanent misery, simply because they have what is described in the medical literature as "subclinical hypothyroidism."

Subclinical hypothyroidism refers to a state in which patients' thyroid hormone levels are too low even though their laboratory results fall within the so-called normal range. A 1983 study published in *Postgraduate Medicine* covered this issue.[1]

In the study, sixty-five women were examined because their many symptoms were suggestive of hypothyroidism. In all cases, the blood tests were within normal range. Using a sophisticated stimulation challenge test, the researchers demonstrated that forty-seven of the women, or a whopping 72 percent, did in fact have hypothyroidism despite the normal test results. So much for the accuracy of standard thyroid hormone screening.

And guess what happened when the researchers treated them with thyroid hormones even though the blood tests were normal? They all improved! Various studies similar to this one have revealed that in any given age group somewhere between 5 and 15 percent of the population has subclinical hypothyroidism. Using Bio-Energy Testing, I have discovered that number to be considerably higher.

Why are the blood tests so unreliable? Well, the most likely reason is that the "normal" reference range for blood tests is based on what is usually found in the general population. And since thyroid deficiency is virtually rampant in the general population, this reference range includes many patients who have demonstrated hypothyroidism. Another reason is that the level of thyroid hormones in the blood can change so rapidly that it is difficult to get an accurate picture of what is going on with only one "snapshot" blood draw.

Bio-Energy Testing to the Rescue

Because testing for thyroid hormone deficiency can be so misleading, physicians aware of subclinical hypothyroidism often have to make the diagnosis simply based on physical examination and clinical symptoms.

One of the great advantages of Bio-Energy Testing is that it is a very sensitive way to determine the presence of low thyroid function, even in cases of subclinical hypothyroidism. This is because Bio-Energy Testing has the capability of determining your energy production while you are at rest. As you will remember from Chapter 2, this is known as your resting metabolic rate, and it is reported on the test as your M-Factor (Metabolic Factor).

The M-Factor directly correlates with thyroid hormone activity, and is able to detect the presence of a deficiency virtually 100 percent of the time. In fact, when the M-Factor is greater than 110, there is no chance that hypothyroidism is present. Similarly, when the M-Factor is less than 90 as it often is, the likelihood of suboptimal thyroid function is very great, even when the thyroid blood tests fail to make the diagnosis.

Using Bio-Energy Testing, I find thyroid hormone deficiency to be present in more than half of my diabetic patients, no matter what their age. When the thyroid hormones are adequately replaced, my patients not only lose fat and have improved energy levels, but they also, not surprisingly, show a much better control of their blood sugar.

Why Are Thyroid Hormones So Often Deficient?

Well, the most common culprit of thyroid hormone deficiency is the very process of aging itself as it relates to the decline in the neuroendocrine axis that I mentioned at the beginning of this chapter. But there are also several other considerations that should be discussed.

For one, there are several environmental factors that can, in effect, poison the thyroid gland. The first one is mercury toxicity. Mercury is selectively toxic to the thyroid gland. Mercury has become ubiquitous in our environment, so much so that many states in America warn pregnant women not to eat the fish caught in the local rivers and lakes because the fish have such a high mercury content. Mercury is extremely harmful to humans in general, but it is particularly damaging in their fetal stage. Recently there have been many headlines in the popular press regarding studies that show elevated mercury levels in people who eat fish on a regular basis.

Also, we should not forget that the scientific literature is loaded with studies that demonstrate that the mercury contained in the dental fillings called "silver amalgams" can leak out of the fillings and collect in the tissues of the body, particularly the thyroid, pituitary, and kidney. This is the most common dental filling material used, and there are very few people who do not have at least one of these fillings.

Another potential environmental cause of hypothyroidism is fluoride. Due to overexposure of fluoride, which is in the water systems and toothpaste, many people develop what is known as fluorosis. One of the signs of fluorosis is white spots on the teeth, something I frequently see in my diabetic patients. Fluoride, though a very important (some even say essential) micromineral for the proper health and function of the veins, arteries, connective tissues, and bones, is toxic to the thyroid in fairly small doses, doses that are often encountered by the general population.

Other factors that can interfere with proper functioning of the thyroid gland are medical, dental, and chiropractic x-rays. All of these exposures occur in very close proximity to the thyroid, which is located in the front of the neck just over the windpipe. A 1993 article on the impact of radiation on the thyroid points out that the thyroid gland "is an organ that is usually susceptible to exposure to ionizing radiation by routine medical examination." The authors then go on to list chest x-rays and dental x-rays as particular culprits, and describe data that "indicates a high incidence of external radiation-induced thyroid tumors as well as hypothyroidism."[2]

Thyroid Hormones and Your Liver

As mentioned earlier, there are two thyroid hormones, T3 and T4. T3 contains three iodine atoms and T4 has four. The fourth iodine on T4 renders it much less active than T3, and so T4 is usually referred to as the inactive form of the hormone. As the active form of the hormone, T3 actually stimulates the cells to produce energy. It is important to know the difference between T3 and T4 in order to understand why the liver is so important to thyroid function: it is in the liver that T4 can be converted to T3.

Ninety-three percent of the hormone that is produced in the thyroid gland and released into circulation in the body is T4, while only 7 percent is T3. Thus, the thyroid supplies the body with just the minimal amount of active hormone that is needed to maintain the basal energy requirements of the resting body. At the same time, by producing so much T4, the thyroid provides the body with an abundance of inactive hormone, which can be converted to T3 in the liver on an as-needed basis.

For example, when your immune system is fighting an infection, and you need a sudden burst of energy to power up your white blood cells, your liver will convert a lot of the circulating T4 into T3, which will then activate your immune response. Similarly, when you exercise and your energy requirements go up, your liver will see to it that you have enough T3 to meet your needs. Obviously, since energy requirements are changing often from minute to minute, the liver plays a very central role in the functioning of the thyroid hormones.

As it turns out, this particular function of the liver is suboptimal in many people, and they are unable to convert T4 to T3 in an efficient manner. Why this occurs is unknown but probably is due to a mixture of liver toxicity, suboptimal nutrition, and genetics. It is also important to note that the elevated levels of cortisol that occur with stress will act to block T4 to T3 conversion.

One of the reasons that thyroid blood tests can miss the diagnosis of thyroid hormone deficiency is that these tests assume that a patient's T4-to-T3 conversion is normal. Fortunately, Bio-Energy Testing takes this conversion into account and will demonstrate the effects of decreased T4-to-T3 conversion during the exercise part of the test. Improved conversion rates can often be attained simply by focusing on therapies that optimize liver function.

Thyroid Hormone Replacement Therapy

Unfortunately, for the most part, conventional physicians do not appreciate how common it is that patients are unable to adequately convert T4 to T3. In fact, they seem to assume that the problem never occurs, and for that reason they not only forget to test for T3 but also often forget to replace it after making a diagnosis of hypothyroidism. This mistake makes it much less probable that they will be offering their patients effective treatments.

It also doesn't make much sense biologically. If the thyroid makes 93 percent T4 and 7 percent T3, you would think that the best way to replace deficient thyroid hormones would be to replace them in this same ratio. Such a ratio can be found in a form of thyroid hormone supplement called desiccated thyroid hormone. Because it comes the closest to mimicking how the thyroid actually functions, I prescribe this form of thyroid hormone replacement in my patients who are deficient. I have seen too many cases of hypothyroid patients who fail to respond optimally when only T4 is being replaced.

CORRECTING CORTISOL IMBALANCE

Cortisol, also known as hydrocortisone, is the principal hormone of the adrenal gland and next to the thyroid hormones is probably the most important single hormone in the body. It is a powerful hormone that is intimately involved in all aspects of metabolism and energy production.

When your body is stressed, whether in the form of worry, fear, or anger or something more tangible like pain, a virus, or an allergy, cortisol is instrumental in making sure that your body handles the stress well. For this reason, it is often known as the "stress hormone."

Gluconeogenesis—Protein to Glucose

From an energy-deficit perspective, cortisol does everything you would want a hormone to do. It increases overall energy production, and it shifts energy production away from glucose metabolism and toward fat metabolism. It does this in several ways, one of which is gluconeogenesis. As discussed earlier, gluconeogenesis refers to the process of converting protein to glucose. Many people erroneously think that it is necessary to eat carbohydrates in order to maintain glucose stores. Actually, because of gluconeogenesis, nothing could be further from the truth.

Earlier in the book I discussed the fact that the ingestion of dietary carbohydrate is a very recent event in human history. What humans have traditionally fed on, and what our systems respond best to, are fat and protein, and cortisol is primarily responsible for our ability to thrive on a protein-and-fat diet.

You will recall that there are only two reasons why we need glucose in the first place, and both of them have to do with emergencies. One is that glucose, unlike fat, can be a source of energy even in the absence of oxygen, and the other is that glucose can supply the faster, more intense forms of energy that are required for emergency escapes, and so on. Therefore, the human body developed the capacity to store glucose in the form of a molecule call glycogen, but since it is only needed for emergencies, the body only evolved the capability of storing a very tiny amount of glycogen.

However, small as they may be, maintaining these glycogen stores is fundamental for human survival and optimum energy output. This is where cortisol comes in. By being the single major stimulator of gluconeogenesis in the body, cortisol causes dietary protein to be converted to glucose and stored as glycogen. As long as your diet contains enough protein and the adrenal glands can maintain adequate cortisol levels, glycogen stores will be maintained and dietary carbohydrate intake is unnecessary.

Cortisol and Fat Metabolism

Cortisol stimulates fat metabolism in two different ways. First, it causes the stored fat in the adipose tissue to be released into circulation so that the cells can take it up for energy. Second, through mechanisms that are not well understood, cortisol actually stimulates the production of energy from fat inside each and every one of the cells.

Because of these two effects, the overall effect of cortisol is to decrease the metabolism of glucose by increasing fat metabolism. It single-handedly is able to correct the metabolic shift that occurs with aging. In this way, cortisol is obviously an extremely important hormone for patients with diabetes.

Cortisol Deficiency

Cortisol deficiency is a close runner-up to the thyroid hormones as the most common hormonal deficiency I see in my patients. They often occur together. In fact, since the cells of the body, including the cells of the adrenal glands, need thyroid hormones in order to function properly, low levels of thyroid hormones often result in the adrenal glands being unable to produce adequate amounts of cortisol.

The most common cause of cortisol deficiency is a diet too high in carbohydrate, especially when it is combined with mental and/or emotional stress. Since these two factors are so predominant in modern-day living, it is no wonder that cortisol deficiency is so widespread. Cortisol deficiency can also result from other chronic stresses such as infection, illness, insomnia, pain, allergies, and so on.

The most classic low-cortisol symptom is fatigue, especially fatigue that worsens in the afternoon. Other common symptoms include allergies, asthma, insomnia, low blood sugar, lightheadedness and fainting, palpitations, difficulty concentrating, attention deficit disorder (ADD), hyperactivity, depression and anxiety, decreased libido, headaches, migraines, backaches, joint aches, and any autoimmune disease. Just to show how common cortisol deficiency is, these symptoms make up more than 95 percent of those I hear all day long in the clinic.

The importance of cortisol and its relationship to chronic stress was first discovered by Hans Selye, M.D., Ph.D., a professor of endocrinology at the University of Montreal. Through his experimentation he made two important observations: first, that the long-term response to stress was mediated by cortisol, and second, that each individual had a genetically predetermined maximum capacity to produce cortisol while under stress. He referred to this capacity as the individual's "adrenal reserve."

This means that when we are exposed to continued stress our adrenal glands begin producing increased amounts of cortisol, which is critical to how well our bodies are able to handle the stress. As the stress continues, the adrenal glands continue to produce elevated amounts of cortisol until one of two possibilities occurs. One, the stress goes away and the adrenal production of cortisol decreases to the pre-stress levels. Two, when the individual's adrenal reserve is exhausted, his adrenal glands will no longer be able to keep producing the elevated amounts of cortisol that his body is demanding, and cortisol levels will decrease even though the stress is still present. At some point, the cortisol levels will become so low that the patient's body can no longer adapt to the stress and it begins to fall apart.

If the patient has the genes for diabetes, it is at this point of low cortisol levels that his or her body will start moving in the direction of the disease. The majority of the patients I see who have been diagnosed with diabetes are in this category, and show a cortisol deficiency when tested.

Cortisol Excess

Dr. Selye also pointed out that since one's adrenal reserve is genetically determined, when two different people are exposed to the same levels of chronic stress, one will break down earlier than the other. He performed many experiments to document this observation. In fact, some people have such an elevated adrenal reserve that they are able to tolerate high stress levels their entire life.

These are the people that can get only five hours of sleep, hardly eat anything at all, drink too much, constantly consume junk food, work like crazy, and yet are able to maintain good energy and mood while never seeming to suffer from anything. They always feel great! Their adrenal glands are able to produce elevated levels of cortisol on an endless basis. Phenotypically, they are usually darker complected, brown-eyed, and male with a mesomorphic build.

People like this suffer from an altogether different kind of problem. They develop disorders that stem from excessive amounts of cortisol, such as elevated cholesterol, heart disease, hypertension, weight gain, and insomnia. Ironically enough, these patients can also develop diabetes because high cortisol levels cause the cell membranes to become resistant to insulin. About 5 percent of the patients I see with diabetes have elevated cortisol levels. The major tip-off that a patient with diabetes may be one who has excessive cortisol is when the patient tells me that he or she feels great and has no symptoms from diabetes.

Testing for Cortisol Deficiency and Excess

One way to test cortisol levels is by examining a fasting blood specimen taken around eight in the morning. The patient should not have exercised or experienced any significant stress, say an argument or a stressful drive to the lab.

The reference range given in most laboratories for cortisol is between 10 and 25 micrograms per deciliter (mcg/dl). However, no level over 15 mcg/dl should be considered acceptable in healthy individuals. I believe that any level over 15 mcg/dl indicates that the body is raising cortisol to unacceptable levels in response to chronic stress.

A better way to assess cortisol is by using a saliva specimen. Saliva is a much more stable specimen than is blood, which is to say that it doesn't vary as much minute by minute, and is often more representative. We will look more closely at the comparative strengths of saliva assays in the next section on DHEA (see "Testing for DHEA Deficiency").

Another good lab test is a twenty-four-hour urine test for free cortisol and for other adrenal metabolites such as DHEA. This test works by measuring how much cortisol was produced over a twenty-four-hour period, and can be very helpful to pinpoint both cortisol deficiency and excess states.

Finally, there is Bio-Energy Testing, which in the presence of adrenal deficiency will show a low M-Factor and, of course, a low Adrenal Factor. I rely on Bio-Energy Testing combined with the patient's symptoms and findings to diagnose the presence of cortisol deficiency. I use the blood, saliva, and urine tests primarily to diagnose cortisol excess.

Treating Cortisol Deficiency: Hormone Replacement Therapy and More

Treating cortisol deficiency is very easy. First of all, be sure to focus on correcting the causes. This usually amounts to decreasing stress and eliminating dietary carbohydrates. In addition to this, cortisol replacement therapy is often very helpful. The hormone can be prescribed by a physician. Although the correct dose can vary enormously from person to person, it is usually 5 to 10 milligrams (mg) taken in the morning and again in the early part of the afternoon.

Other very helpful treatments that I use all the time are licorice extract, which acts on the liver to help maintain cortisol levels, and capsules of liver and adrenal extract, vitamin C, and the B vitamin pantothenic acid. These are over-the-counter supplements easily obtained at any health food store and they are discussed in Chapter 7. Although they can usually be safely taken according to the instructions on the label, I would strongly recommend that you be guided by a physician knowledgeable about nutritional and herbal therapies before you start self-medicating.

Treating Cortisol Excess

Treating cortisol excess is not always so easy as treating a deficiency. Patients with this problem are not usually all that well motivated to make changes. Since they typically feel great, they can't see why their lifestyle and the way they view life need to be overhauled. They need to be encouraged to decrease their levels of stress and eliminate carbohydrates from their diet.

In addition, fifteen minutes of meditation in the morning and again in the evening will almost always significantly help improve cortisol excess. The problem here is that people with high cortisol usually have type-A personalities and are so driven that they have a hard time sitting around doing nothing. Even though meditation is not "doing nothing," that is how it is often perceived, and it is often very hard to get these patients to discipline themselves to do it. If they are willing to give meditation a try, however, it will often turn their clinical condition completely around.

CORRECTING DHEA IMBALANCE

Of all of the steroid hormones in the body, including cortisol, the estrogens, and testosterone, DHEA is the most abundant. Of the hundreds of clinical and scientific papers on DHEA, many repeatedly point to several very dramatic physiological and medical effects from supplementation of this hormone. These effects include the following:

- Protecting the immune system against infections of all types.

- Decreasing the incidence of virtually all diseases of aging, such as cancer, heart disease, osteoporosis, and arthritis.

- Preventing and treating chronic depression, learning disabilities, and memory loss.

- Controlling autoimmune diseases such as lupus and rheumatoid arthritis.

- Improving energy production from both fat and sugar metabolism.

Of course, by now you will recognize that this last energy-enhancing property of DHEA makes it a prime candidate for the diabetes hormone-of-the-month club.

DHEA is a hormone that, like cortisol, is produced in the adrenal glands. It is often deficient in conditions that deplete the adrenal glands, such as aging, chronic stress, illness, pain, insomnia, and so on. It has been labeled "the mother of all hormones" because it has the ability to be converted in the body to estrogen, testosterone, progesterone, and even cortisol on an as-needed basis. Because of this potential ability to regulate all steroid hormones, as I doctor I consider it to be one of the most important hormones I can replace, and I rarely prescribe any hormone replacement without first looking at DHEA levels.

According to Dr. Ronald Klatz, president of the American Academy of Anti-Aging Medicine, by the age of seventy-five, DHEA levels are only 10 to 20 percent of what they were at age twenty.[3] But though DHEA, for this reason and for all of the other reasons already mentioned, is usually thought of as an anti-aging hormone, I think of it primarily as an antidiabetes hormone because of its demonstrated capacity to prevent diabetes even in genetically predisposed animals, increase fat metabolism, and increase insulin sensitivity.

DHEA and Diabetes Prevention

Since preventing a disease is infinitely better than treating it, let's first take a look at the ability of DHEA to prevent diabetes. And here we meet an interesting dilemma regarding prevention studies in humans.

Due to the fact that humans live so long, it would take a minimum of twenty years to finish any kind of study that would demonstrate whether or not DHEA replacement could prevent diabetes. This is just way too long of a wait to learn about such a potentially important intervention. But such a time problem is obviated when the research is conducted on animals with much shorter life spans, and is why researchers look to animal studies to give us an idea of what is likely to happen with humans.

One of the many animal studies that demonstrate the diabetes-preventing effect of DHEA was published over twenty years ago in the journal *Diabetes*. In this 1984 study, mice that were genetically bred to become obese and develop diabetes were treated with DHEA added to their diet.

When the DHEA was added early on, at the age of two weeks, the researchers found that the treatment "prevented the development of most diabetes symptoms and decreased the rate of weight gain."[4] Remember now that these were not regular mice. Under usual circumstances, 100 percent of these mice develop diabetes. That DHEA had this effect in these particular mice was very remarkable.

Even when the DHEA was not added to the diet until very late, at the age of two years, the mice still demonstrated "improved glucose tolerance," while at the same time their insulin levels were reduced to "younger" levels. Amazingly, according to the findings in this study, "DHEA prevented hyperglycemia [high blood sugar], islet cell atrophy [the destruction of the cells that make insulin], and severe diabetes"[5]—in this group of mice who were inbred to develop *all* of these conditions.

DHEA and Fat Metabolism

Like its biochemically related brother, testosterone, DHEA has been shown to have the effect of increasing muscle mass while at the same time decreasing fat stores.

Examples of this effect can be found in several statistical studies that show that obese patients almost always have much lower circulating levels of DHEA than non-obese subjects. Additionally, other studies have proven DHEA to be very effective at mediating weight loss due to its ability to increase energy production specifically from fat.

For example, in one study DHEA was administered to thirty middle-aged men and women for eight weeks in conjunction with a 1,800 calorie daily diet and one hour of exercise per day. Another group of matched subjects were given the diet and the exercise without the DHEA supplementation. Impressively, those subjects receiving the DHEA lost more than three times the amount of weight than the non-DHEA group.[6]

According to a review article published in the *International Journal of Obesity* on the role of DHEA in energy production, DHEA has been shown to stimulate the body's resting energy production by increasing the metabolism of fat. Sounds like a great idea to me! Not only that, but the article also points out that through its effects on the cells' insulin receptors, DHEA also makes the cell more sensitive to insulin.[7]

The fat-metabolizing effects of DHEA are also underscored in an interesting and unusual article that found that postmenopausal females who applied a 10 percent topical DHEA cream to their skin on a daily basis for one year experienced a 9.8 percent decrease in their quantity of subcutaneous fat and a 3.8 percent decrease in femoral fat.[8]

Another very extraordinary study looked at the effect of DHEA supplementation in fifty-six elderly men and women between the ages of sixty-five and seventy-eight years, all of whom had age-related decreases in their blood DHEA levels. For six months, half of the group received DHEA and the other half received a placebo. No other measures to reduce weight were initiated. Using magnetic resonance imaging (MRI), the researchers were literally able to measure the volume of fat found in the subcutaneous tissues as well as in the abdomen.

It must have been pretty easy for those researchers to guess which patients were on the DHEA and which were on the placebo because at the end of the study period, those on DHEA had lost about three times as much fat as the patients on the placebo had gained! The authors concluded, "DHEA replacement could play a role in the prevention and treatment of the metabolic syndrome associated with abdominal obesity."[9]

Keep in mind that the metabolic syndrome is one of the first steps on the road that leads to diabetes.

DHEA and Insulin Sensitivity

For over sixty years it has been recognized that normal human aging is associated with a progressive loss of insulin sensitivity. This fact is one of the major reasons why the risk of developing diabetes steadily increases each year that we get older. The fact that aging is also associated with a similar decrease in DHEA production is probably not simple coincidence. Therefore, it should not be too surprising to any student of DHEA that replacing deficient DHEA levels in aging patients has been shown to improve insulin sensitivity.

In one study published in 2003, twenty-four middle-aged men were given either DHEA or a placebo for three months. The researchers examined whether or not insulin sensitivity was affected by the DHEA supplementation. They concluded, "Taken together, our results indicate that long-term DHEA supplementation may assist in maintaining optimal insulin sensitivity."[10]

We have already looked at the fact that underactive adrenal glands often play a big role in the genesis of diabetes in certain patients. Therefore, since DHEA is the most abundant hormone produced in the adrenals, it is not surprising that one group of researchers actively looked at what happens to insulin sensitivity when a group of patients with known adrenal insufficiency supplements with DHEA. They concluded that "replacement therapy with 50 mg DHEA for 12 weeks significantly increased insulin sensitivity in hypoadrenal women, thereby suggesting that DHEA replacement could have a potential impact in preventing type 2 diabetes."[11]

Testing for DHEA Deficiency

The easiest and most economical way to test DHEA levels is to use a saliva specimen. Blood can also be used, but blood is just not the best specimen for the analysis of most hormones. There are two reasons for this.

First, blood levels do not discriminate between hormones that are free or "unbound" and those that are bound to proteins. This is important because hormones that are bound to proteins cannot exert their effect; thus, measuring them can be very misleading.

Secondly, the levels of most hormones in the bloodstream can fluctuate so fast that it is hard to get an idea of what the steady-state level of a hormone is simply by looking at one blood specimen. In fact, the only accurate way to examine the levels of hormones from a blood specimen is to perform three blood draws, each twenty to thirty minutes apart, and then mix all three specimens together before sending them to the lab. This is a great way to enhance accuracy, but I know of very few physicians and patients alike who have the patience to undergo such measures.

Saliva hormone assays have neither of these drawbacks. Saliva assays only measure free or unbound hormones, and the levels are remarkably steady from hour to hour. Various laboratories may use different analyzing techniques so it is not possible to give you what the statistical range is, since it may vary from lab to lab. Suffice it to say that I always use the same laboratory, and I like my patients to have levels greater than the middle range shown on the lab test result. If it is lower than that range, I will consider supplementing with DHEA.

DHEA Replacement Therapy

A good way to start improving DHEA levels naturally is to exercise. It is possible to double your DHEA levels for the day simply by exercising for twenty minutes.

Similarly, DHEA levels can be increased by avoiding dietary carbohydrates. This is because carbohydrates result in increases in insulin, and insulin has been shown to block the synthesis of DHEA in the adrenal glands. Here is yet one more reason to add to the ever-growing list of why we need to keep a lid on our carbohydrate intake.

In terms of supplementing with DHEA, typical doses are as follows: for men, about 25–50 mg per day; for women, about 10–25 mg per day. At these doses, I rarely encounter side effects in men, but it is important to note that about one in every twenty women will report either hair loss or oily skin often associated with acne. Fortunately when this occurs, a reduction in the dose will eliminate the problem.

Caution: Remember that earlier I pointed out that DHEA is often called the "mother of all hormones" because it has the potential to be turned into other hormones such as estrogen and testosterone? So, DHEA very often will increase the levels of both of these hormones, and this bears a word of caution regarding the use of supplementary DHEA. First of all, it should never be used in a patient with either breast or prostate cancer, because both of these cancers grow more rapidly in the presence of either the estrogens or testosterone. Any man or woman taking DHEA should do so only under the advice of a physician, and only after being properly screened for the presence of breast and prostate cancer. Secondly, in men over the age of fifty, close to 35 percent will experience elevated estrogen levels as a result of supplementing with doses of DHEA over 50 mg per day. Occasionally, even smaller doses can have this effect. Although estrogen is a great hormone for women, in men it can cause problems such as impotence and prostate swelling. Therefore, any man taking DHEA should not only have his DHEA levels followed up, but also his estrogen levels.

In summary, when properly used, DHEA is easily one of the most valuable tools we have not only in the prevention of diabetes and obesity, but also in the treatment of the two related conditions.

CORRECTING TESTOSTERONE IMBALANCE

Over the years I have found that a deficiency of testosterone is not only common in patients with diabetes, particularly men, but in fact it is the rule. This is not particularly surprising since testosterone is very much involved in increasing energy production, as well as improving fat metabolism.

I learned early on that my patients showed a significant improvement in their diabetes after replacing deficient testosterone. Many patients who had found it impossible to control their blood sugars would show non-diabetes blood glucose levels once they had their testosterone levels normalized.

A number of research studies are starting to demonstrate this remarkable relationship between blood sugar and testosterone levels. For example, in the results of a study published in 2003 in the journal *Aging Male*, the researchers reported what happened when they supplemented twenty-four type 2 diabetic men with testosterone therapy for only three months. They then compared the results with another twenty-four men with type 2 diabetes who did not receive testosterone. What they found was that the men who received testosterone replacement had a 20 percent improvement in their blood sugar control despite the fact that testosterone was the only additional form of treatment used.[12]

More important for me, since I am just as interested in preventing diabetes as I am in treating it, is another study of 1,709 men that appeared in *Diabetes Care* in 2000. In this study, the testosterone levels of the participants were measured, and then the men were followed up for seven to ten years to see if there was any relationship between low testosterone levels and the development of diabetes. At the end of the study, the men with the lowest levels of testosterone were close to two times more likely to have developed diabetes than those with the highest levels. The authors made the following observation: "The results of the present study are consistent with other reports that low levels of SHBG [sex hormone binding globulin] and testosterone play a role in the development of insulin resistance and subsequently the development of type 2 diabetes."[13]

There are quite a few studies like this that report similar results and demonstrate that many cases of diabetes can be completely prevented by replacing deficient testosterone levels when they are present. By the way, this study also points out an important relationship between the thyroid hormone T3, testosterone levels, and diabetes, since it is a deficiency of T3 that causes a decrease in SHBG.

Testing for Testosterone Deficiency

The best way to diagnose testosterone deficiency is by the presence of the symptoms. These are weight gain, fatigue, decreased stamina, depression, apathy, diminished libido, erectile dysfunction, loss of leg hair, and breast development in men. In Bio-Energy Testing the finding is a decreased Fitness Factor. It is important to mention here that testosterone deficiency is just as common in women, and just as important to treat in women as it is in men.

The most sensitive blood test measures the free testosterone level at around eight in the morning. Because of the minute-to-minute variation in blood testosterone levels, it is recommended that three different blood samples be taken twenty minutes apart. These specimens are then all mixed together and sent to the lab as one specimen.

As important as the testosterone level is the estradiol level in a man. Estradiol is an estrogen, but the male body also makes it by converting testosterone into estradiol. This conversion is accomplished by an enzyme called aromatase, which is normally held in check by T3. Unfortunately, due to the low levels of T3 that are so common in the over-fifty age group, the enzyme aromatase increases its activity, which results in higher estradiol levels and lower testosterone levels.

Thus, when ordering a free-testosterone-level test, it is also important to evaluate estradiol and SHBG as well. Low levels of SHBG are a reliable indicator of low levels of T3. If the testosterone and the SHBG levels are toward the lower end of their reference ranges, and the estradiol is toward the upper end of its range, then it is likely that the patient has a combination of both T3 and testosterone deficiency.

I always get lab tests to determine testosterone levels, but because the reference range is so large, if the patient has enough of the symptoms, I will prescribe a therapeutic trial even if the test results are within range. In a therapeutic trial, I will administer testosterone replacement therapy for about three months in order to observe whether or not the patient's symptoms improve.

Testosterone Replacement Therapy

There are a number of ways testosterone can be replaced, and they all have their relative advantages and disadvantages. Unfortunately, testosterone is not absorbed well when taken orally, so it either has to be taken transdermally as a patch or a topical cream or gel, or it can be administered as an injection.

When an injection is used, it can either be injected intramuscularly one to two times per week or injected as a pellet implant every one to two months. The intramuscular injections are usually done in the physician's office, but many of my patients have learned to inject themselves at home. The pellet implants, on the other hand, can only be done in the doctor's office. I tend to use testosterone replacement therapy in the following way: I prescribe an intramuscular injection twice a week for three months to establish therapeutic levels, and then switch the patient over to a topical cream for long-term maintenance.

An alternative way to increase testosterone levels is by taking androstenedione and/or DHEA capsules. These two adrenal hormones are converted in the body to testosterone, and can often be a very effective way to treat testosterone deficiency, especially in women. They have the advantage of being much less expensive than testosterone, and can be taken orally. The problem that is frequently encountered with them when they are used to treat men is that they can also be converted to estradiol. In fact, in many men these hormones will increase estradiol levels more than they increase testosterone levels, thus rendering the treatment ineffective.

Whatever way the physician decides to treat testosterone deficiency, it is always important to regularly monitor both the testosterone and the estradiol levels until they are stabilized on a known dose. Additionally, in men it is important to carefully monitor the effects of the treatments on the prostate. This means the physician needs to make an initial prostate examination as well as do a PSA (prostate-specific antigen) test for signs of prostate cancer every three months for the first year on therapy.

These precautions should be taken because both testosterone and estradiol stimulate prostate growth, and if the man being treated happens to have an undiagnosed prostate cancer, replacing his testosterone levels will cause the cancer to grow faster. This can easily be determined by noticing an increase in the PSA levels during treatment. If the PSA levels are found to increase, then the best choice is to avoid the use of testosterone, as it is too risky to persist.

If during testosterone replacement the physician notices that the estradiol levels are increasing due to the conversion activity of aromatase, he or she can prescribe one of two treatments. The first is an herbal remedy called chrysin. Chrysin is an extract of the passionflower plant, which in many cases is able to significantly decrease aromatase activity. The second is medication that acts as an aromatase inhibitor, which is easily available by prescription and very safe to use.

CORRECTING GROWTH HORMONE IMBALANCE

Growth hormone is a hormone that is made in the brain in large amounts when we are young, and declines steadily as we get older. It is called growth hormone because of its stimulating effects on the growth plates of growing bones. As will be discussed in this section, growth hormone also has several other important effects. It has a positive effect on fat metabolism, it stimulates the growth of muscle and bone cells, and it causes the liver to produce insulinlike growth factor 1 (IGF-1).

Because growth hormone is so fundamental for stimulating the growth of bones, a deficiency of growth hormone in children results in short stature because it results in insufficient bone growth. Similarly, in adults, even though their period of bone growth ended in the teenage years, a deficiency results in osteoporosis because growth hormone is essential to maintaining optimal bone status. The resultant osteoporosis from adult-onset growth hormone deficiency is what is responsible for the loss of height seen in aging persons.

Common symptoms and clinical signs of growth hormone deficiency are as follows:

- Decreased energy

- Mood disturbances

- Reduced vitality

- Reduced exercise stamina and performance

- Impotence

- Reduced libido

- Decreased quality of sleep

- Decreased memory

- Decreased ability to focus and concentrate

- Osteoporosis

- Muscle loss and weakness

- Obesity

- Decreased HDL cholesterol (the "good" cholesterol)

- Increased LDL cholesterol (the "bad" cholesterol)

- Decreased metabolic rate (M-Factor in Bio-Energy Testing)

- Decreased anaerobic threshold (EQ in Bio-Energy Testing)

- Decreased fat metabolism (C-Factor and Fat-Burning Factor in Bio-Energy Testing)

- Sagging muscles (especially on the back of arms and buttocks)

- Sagging facial muscles (that is, the jowls)

- Decreased hair growth

- Congestive heart failure

- Decreased wound healing

- Thinning skin

While decreased growth hormone levels are an inevitable part of the aging process, there are several ways you can boost sagging levels. As will be discussed, these include lifestyle factors such as exercise and hormone replacement.

The Anti-Fat Hormone

Growth hormone has a powerful action on fat metabolism called lipolysis, which causes fat cells to release their fat content for energy production. You might remember that thyroid hormone also shares this effect, and there is evidence that growth hormone assists thyroid hormone in this action. Without lipolysis, your body would be unable to burn fat, and it would just accumulate in the fat cells. Sound familiar?

Because of growth hormone's importance in lipolysis, a deficiency may be a major factor in the development of obesity. This is dramatically illustrated by the marked difference between growth hormone levels in obese men and those in normal men. Whereas non-obese men produce 540 ± 44 micrograms of growth hormone over a twenty-four-hour period, obese men only produce 77 ± 20 micrograms, only a fraction of what is required to adequately metabolize fat.[14]

As you have already seen, decreased fat metabolism is one of the major reasons we develop an energy deficit as we get older, which in turn is the major cause of type 2 diabetes. Furthermore, the obesity that ultimately develops as a result of decreased fat metabolism is itself the single major cause of type 2 diabetes. When adults with growth hormone deficiency have their sagging levels replaced, they lose an average of about 15 percent of their body fat mass.

The Muscle/Bone Hormone

Growth hormone also stimulates muscle and bone cells to grow and multiply. Patients who are deficient in growth hormone end up losing significant amounts of their muscle and bone mass. In medical terms this combined loss is referred to as a loss of lean body mass. The degree of loss can be dramatic. Using Bio-Energy Testing (remember that functional muscle mass can be determined by the Fitness Factor), I often see patients who are only in their fifties who have lost more than 50 percent of their functional muscle mass! Deficient muscle mass, in turn, aggravates insulin resistance, raising blood sugars and further setting the stage for type 2 diabetes. When adults with growth hormone deficiency are properly treated, they gain back an average of about 10 percent of their lean fat mass.

The Antidiabetic Hormone

Finally, growth hormone stimulates the liver to produce another very powerful hormone with a considerably less colorful name, insulinlike growth factor 1, or IGF-1 for short. IGF-1 activates the insulin receptors in the body, leading to increased insulin sensitivity and decreased insulin levels. So in essence, IGF-1 is an antidiabetic hormone!

Not surprisingly, although it is not yet commercially available, when given to both type 2 and type 1 diabetics, IGF-1 reverses many of the signs and symptoms of diabetes. I believe that decreased IGF-1 levels caused by growth hormone deficiency is one of the major factors leading to type 2 diabetes in genetically susceptible people.

How to Boost Sagging Growth Hormone Levels

Remember that developing a deficiency of growth hormone as you get older is inevitable. It is just as predictable as developing deficiencies in all of your other hormones. It's not a question of if, but rather of when. Therefore, as you become deficient in growth hormone, you will very gradually become shorter, develop osteoporosis, lose muscle mass and replace it with fat, and become less sensitive to insulin and more prone to type 2 diabetes. By the time you or your friends actually see it, these problems may already have progressed much further than desirable. You will also slowly but surely develop many of the common symptoms and clinical signs of growth hormone deficiency, as listed at the beginning of this section.

What is not so certain is when you can expect growth hormone levels to reach deficient levels. In my case it happened in my late forties, but in others it arrives much earlier or later. Very clearly, both genetics and the very process of aging itself are the major factors in causing growth hormone deficiency, but there are also some lifestyle factors that have a significant effect on growth hormone production.

Exercise

As remarkable as it may sound, simply exercising for as little as twenty minutes, in many cases, will double growth hormone levels for the day. Twenty minutes of exercise may not sound like much, but it is when you consider that the majority of the adult population at risk of diabetes has no exercise routine at all.

Sleep

Growth hormone is made in a part of the brain called the pituitary during stage 3 and stage 4 sleep. These are the deepest stages of sleep. You can simply observe when someone is sleeping in these deeper levels of sleep because it becomes much harder to wake them up, even with fairly loud noises. Likewise, when you are suddenly awakened out of stage 4 sleep, as I am occasionally for some medical emergency, for several minutes you feel as though you are drugged.

For a variety of reasons, many people simply don't get enough stage 3 and stage 4 sleep, and as a result, their production of growth hormone can be dramatically decreased. Studies have demonstrated that the loss of only four hours of sleep will produce diabetic glucose tolerance patterns in healthy young men in only five days.

Diet

It has been well established that fasting for as little as ten hours will increase growth hormone levels significantly, enough to increase fat metabolism and improve blood sugar maintenance. In fact, short periods of abstinence are much more effective in this regard than longer periods, because although prolonged fasting increases growth hormone production, it also results in decreased IGF-1. And decreased IGF-1 levels offset many of the positive effects of growth hormone.

Since not eating for several hours tends to have a favorable influence on growth hormone production, it should not be too surprising that eating frequently has the opposite effect. In this day of twenty-four-hour food availability, it is easy to forget that our metabolisms developed in an environment in which food was not readily available. The practice of "grazing" during the day that has been promoted by some nutritionists is not natural and does not follow the logic of our evolved metabolisms. Furthermore, it results in lowered growth hormone levels, decreased fat metabolism, obesity, and ultimately type 2 diabetes.

So by just avoiding the dangerous myth of eating three squares a day, you can automatically increase your levels of growth hormone, and avoid the vicious cycle of frequent eating that leads to decreased fat metabolism that leads to decreased energy production that leads to increased hunger that leads to eating frequently—while all the time gaining weight and increasing diabetes risk. In this regard I often advise my patients whether they are diabetic or not, to avoid breakfast at least four or five days out of the week. This simple measure results in a fourteen- to sixteen-hour fasting period, which can substantially increase growth hormone output. Remember that as long as diabetics insure that their liver function is optimal they do great on fasts, and those taking insulin will need to adjust their doses accordingly.

The composition of the diet is also important. A diet high in protein increases both growth hormone and IGF-1 levels. Conversely, a diet high in carbohydrates, particularly those carbohydrates high on the glycemic index, results in lower levels of both of these hormones. So, your growth hormone and IGF-1 levels are yet another important reason for you to shift your diet in the direction of protein and away from carbohydrate.

When you consider the sum total of the exercise, sleeping, and eating habits of the average American, it is not hard to understand how decreased levels of growth hormone production have come to be such a significant factor in our diabetes epidemic.

Testing for Growth Hormone Deficiency

As with many of the hormones, testing for growth hormone deficiency is a little bit less than perfect. Perhaps the best overall test is a blood test for IGF-1.

Although IGF-1 levels are not actually a measurement of growth hormone itself, they can serve as an indicator of growth hormone activity, because IGF-1 is formed in the liver in response to the presence of growth hormone. Most physicians are like me and prefer to use IGF-1 as a test for growth hormone, because many if not most of the benefits of growth hormone stem not from the hormone itself but from IGF-1. Additionally, it should be noted that the direct measurement of growth hormone itself is difficult, expensive, sometimes dangerous, and often inaccurate.

In adults, IGF-1 levels significantly decrease with age, so much so that the values in the average seventy-year-old man are less than half of what they were when he was thirty-five. Happily enough, however, when he is treated with growth hormone, studies show that it is quite possible to restore these depleted IGF-1 levels to those common of youth. There is, therefore, strong evidence that the decline we see in IGF-1 with increasing age is, in fact, a result of declining growth hormone levels, and that checking IGF-1 levels is the best way to both diagnose growth hormone deficiency and monitor growth hormone replacement therapy.

As you can imagine, the values for IGF-1 blood levels vary enormously due to genetic and lifestyle factors, so most physicians use the level of 230 nanograms per milliliter (ng/ml) to signify the onset of growth hormone deficiency. This level is the median level that is found in normal healthy subjects between the ages of twenty-six and sixty-seven. IGF-1 levels lower than this are likely to reflect growth hormone deficiency.

In the end, if a given patient has an IGF-1 level of less than 230 ng/ml and also has some of the signs and symptoms of growth hormone deficiency, the only way to be sure of such a deficiency is to perform a clinical trial. A clinical trial means administering growth hormone for three to six months and observing what happens. A diagnosis of growth hormone deficiency is then confirmed when growth hormone replacement therapy results in a significant increase in IGF-1 levels along with a clinical improvement in the patient.

Growth Hormone Replacement Therapy

I love growth hormone! I believe it is the single most powerful hormone we can use to combat the aging process and prevent diabetes. However, there are two significant potential limitations. One is that it is quite expensive, and a course of complete replacement can cost in excess of $200 per month. Fortunately, this problem can be offset simply by using it less often. Studies have shown that even when growth hormone is replaced for only one week out of the month, there is still a significantly positive overall effect.

The other possible drawback is that when it is used to treat a diabetic, growth hormone may initially worsen blood sugar control. It does this because at high enough doses, it has an anti-insulin effect, which acts to increase insulin resistance. The increased insulin resistance results in a compensatory increase in insulin levels combined with an elevation of blood sugar levels. Just what we don't want! This effect has been so widely studied and publicized that many physicians who routinely use growth hormone therapy in their nondiabetic patients are afraid to use it in their diabetic patients. However, this problem turns out to be dose related.

For example, daily doses greater than 6.0 micrograms per kilogram (ug/kg) have been shown to routinely result in increased insulin resistance and higher blood sugars. On the other hand, more physiological dosing (that is, dosing that is in line with the amount that is normally present in the body) such as 2.5–5.0 ug/kg per day has provided satisfactory clinical improvements, combined with optimum IGF-1 levels and a lack of any negative consequences.[15]

Furthermore, the anti-insulin effect of growth hormone tends to be less and less of a problem with time because of its other positive effects, such as fat loss, increased muscle mass, and increased IGF-1 levels. All in all, when I treat a type 2 diabetes patient with proper growth hormone dosing, in combination with other measures you have been learning about in this book, I very rarely find that it does anything other than bring about noticeable clinical improvement.

The best times to self-administer growth hormone injections are before bedtime and again in the morning. It is administered as a subcutaneous injection. This is the same kind of injection that diabetics use for insulin, and in fact we use the exact same kind of needle and syringe. It is an *extremely easy and painless* injection that anyone can give themselves.

When I decide to treat a diabetic patient with growth hormone, I always follow a two-point plan. First, I only start with the smallest dose necessary to improve the IGF-1 level. I decide on how low a dose to use based upon the patient's insulin levels. In a patient with higher insulin levels, I start with lower doses, because such a patient is at a greater risk of developing a significant increase in insulin resistance. Then, while regularly monitoring insulin levels and blood sugar, I will gradually increase the dose over a six-month interval until I get the desired IGF-1 level. If at any time I notice rising blood sugar or insulin levels, I will decrease the dose and then advance at a slower pace. Using this cautious technique I have been able to provide many of my patients all of the advantages of growth hormone replacement without any negative effects on blood sugar control.

What Else Can Help?

Obviously, it would be a little ridiculous to administer growth hormone replacement or, for that matter, to even attempt to diagnose growth hormone deficiency in a patient without at least insuring that he or she is covering the basics with healthy lifestyle choices. That means getting adequate sleep, routinely exercising, and maintaining a high protein, low-carbohydrate diet. Only once these measures have been fully adopted for several months, is it practical to obtain an IGF-1 level. If it turns out to be low, then and only then should growth hormone replacement be administered.

Additionally, especially in my patients who are younger than fifty, IGF-1 levels can be raised significantly by supplementing with certain protein constituents called amino acids. Amino acids should be taken on an empty stomach before bedtime. There are a number of amino acid combinations that you can purchase at the health food store that have been shown to raise IGF-1 levels, but the ones that seem to work the best in my patients are L-glutamine and ornithine ketoglutarate.

I have the patient take the following before bedtime: 2,000 mg of L-glutamine, 1,800 mg of ornithine ketoglutarate, 300 mg of niacin, and 3 ounces of fruit juice. The niacin and the fruit juice enhance the effect of the amino acids. I have seen this particular combination literally double the production of growth hormone in many of my younger patients with type 2 diabetes.

In summary, when growth hormone is looked at simply from the perspective of what it is capable of doing, it sounds like the ultimate prescription for preventing and treating diabetes. For example, it affects the individual's energy dynamics in such a way as to increase fat metabolism while at the same time increasing metabolic rate and lean body mass formation. Not only that, but it also stimulates the liver to produce more IGF-1, a hormone that simultaneously increases insulin sensitivity and decreases insulin levels.

And as you have seen, increasing growth hormone levels is just one more reason why we should all strive to eat, sleep, and exercise better. Of course, it should be used with caution, but my experience has shown me that when judiciously used in combination with a comprehensive and total program to improve energy production, growth hormone replacement often provides the missing link needed for optimum success in both the prevention and treatment of type 2 diabetes.

CHAPTER 13

STEP EIGHT:
Oxidative Medicine, or "Exercise in a Bottle"

One of the first duties of the physician
is to educate the masses not to take medicine.
—SIR WILLIAM OSLER, PHYSICIAN,
CONSIDERED TO BE THE FATHER OF MODERN MEDICINE (1849–1919)

Some patients come to me with more advanced diabetes and can't exercise properly, and so, it's necessary to help them improve to a point where they can add exercise to their treatment program. To achieve this, I use oxidative medicine, or what I have come to refer to as "exercise in a bottle."

WHAT OXIDATIVE MEDICINE IS

The first thing to point out about oxidative medicine is that it is not the same as simply administering oxygen. It does not supply more oxygen to the body. Thus, though the substances used in oxidative medicine do contain molecular oxygen, the process is not simply about getting more oxygen into the tissues. Just getting more oxygen in your body is easily handled by the direct administration of oxygen, a practice common in hospitals around the world. In these cases, oxygen is given to patients who don't have enough oxygen, usually as a result of lung or heart disease, and the oxygen is used simply to fill an oxygen debt.

Oxidative medicine is quite different because we use it not in patients who are lacking oxygen, but in patients who, though they may have sufficient levels of oxygen in their bodies, are unable to utilize it well because of poor mitochondrial function. As a result, their bodies suffer from decreased energy production. Administering oxygen to a person with decreased oxygen utilization would be about as effective as pumping more gas into an inefficient automobile engine.

Oxidative medicine improves oxygen utilization through the administration of hydrogen peroxide or ozone, both of which are biochemically classified as very strong oxidants. An oxidant is a molecule that has such a strong need for electrons, it will pull electrons from other molecules. When it does this, it sets off a series of reactions referred to as oxidative reactions. It is these oxidative reactions that are critically involved in the ways in which our cells utilize oxygen. Thus, to use our engine metaphor, oxidative medicine does to your cells what a tune-up and a new set of spark plugs does for your car: it improves the efficiency with which your cells can metabolize oxygen into energy.

It is important to note that not every molecule that contains oxygen is an oxidant. Consider water for example. Water contains two hydrogen atoms combined with one oxygen atom, but it has no oxidant potential at all. Inject water into someone and nothing happens. However, once another oxygen atom is added to a water molecule, the compound hydrogen peroxide is formed. Hydrogen peroxide is made up of two hydrogen atoms and two oxygen atoms, and that extra oxygen atom makes it a very strong oxidant. Hydrogen peroxide is, therefore, one of the most common molecules used in oxidative medicine.

Another example can be found in the molecule of oxygen itself. An oxygen molecule, which consists of two oxygen atoms, is a strong oxidant. But because it is relatively stable in its two-atom configuration, it is not useful for oxidative medicine. Add another oxygen atom to an oxygen molecule, however, and you form the compound ozone, which has three oxygen atoms instead of the two found in oxygen. Once again, the presence of that extra oxygen atom turns oxygen into one of the strongest oxidants in all of Nature.

Thus, oxidative medicine consists of the administration of either hydrogen peroxide or ozone into the blood. Of course, being strong oxidants, these molecules can be quite damaging if not used correctly, and so physicians must first learn the indications, contraindications, and technique of administration before using them to treat diabetes.

When used correctly in the appropriate patient, especially as part of a complete comprehensive program for diabetes, the effects of oxidative medicine are often dramatic: it helps to improve the delivery of oxygen to the cells, and once the oxygen is there it helps the cells to produce more energy from the oxygen they get. The net result is a rather marked increase in energy production.

HOW OXIDATIVE MEDICINE CAN HELP DIABETICS

Let's start with our old friend 2,3 DPG. You may remember from Chapter 7 that it is 2,3 DPG that causes your blood's hemoglobin molecule to release the oxygen it is carrying and deposit it in the cells. In this way 2,3 DPG plays a very central role in energy production, because without it all the cells would become deprived of oxygen, even when there is plenty of oxygen in the blood.

Research shows that the blood of those with diabetes contains much less 2,3 DPG than those who do not have the disorder, which is certainly one of the reasons why diabetics produce so much less energy. Like most mechanisms in the body, 2,3 DPG is activated by an oxidative reaction; therefore, 2,3 DPG levels can be restored to normal, even in those with diabetes, by using oxidative medicine.

Another way oxidative medicine can be helpful has to do with fat metabolism. Fat metabolism is directly related to the ratio of a niacin molecule called NADH to its oxidized version called NAD. In order for fats to be efficiently metabolized there must be a sufficiently low ratio of NADH to NAD. Due to inadequate oxygen utilization, those with diabetes often do not have a low enough ratio. Oxidants such as hydrogen peroxide and ozone are able to oxidize NADH into NAD and thus lower the ratio, paving the way to more efficient fat burning.

Still another way oxidative medicine can be useful in diabetes is at the cellular receptor sites for insulin. Not surprisingly, it turns out that the biochemical mechanisms that allow insulin to activate these receptor sites are dependent on oxidative reactions. Thus, administering oxidative medicine results in an improved ability of insulin to function through the receptors, which in turn translates to improved insulin sensitivity. In this way, oxidative medicine cuts to the very core of the primary pathology behind diabetes.

Finally, the last area involved in the improvement of diabetes with oxidative medicine is in the mitochondria themselves. As you probably already know by now, mitochondria are the precise areas in the cells where oxygen is metabolized into energy. I have already mentioned the two vital elements for energy production in the mitochondria, the Krebs cycle and the electron transfer system.

The Krebs cycle, which supplies the electron transfer system with hydrogen atoms, is similar to fat metabolism in that it is also controlled by the ratio of NADH to NAD. When this ratio is not sufficiently low, as is often the case in diabetes, the Krebs cycle slows down and is not able to adequately supply hydrogen to the electron transfer system. This, in effect, shuts down energy production. Oxidative medicine improves the ratio and solves the problem.

Whether it is through the increase in 2,3 DPG levels, enhanced fat metabolism, increased insulin sensitivity, improved Krebs cycle function, or any combination of the above, the research is quite clear: the administration of oxidative medicine to any subject with diabetes increases energy production. From a clinical standpoint, these safe, simple, and inexpensive therapies are very effective in treating diabetes, even far-advanced diabetes.

I particularly find oxidative medicine to be helpful in any of the following conditions: (1) diabetes with poor or erratic control of blood sugar, a condition often referred to as brittle diabetes; (2) the presence of any of the complications of diabetes such as cardiovascular disease, retinopathy, decreased kidney function, decreased vision, or gangrene; and (3) when a person with diabetes is unable to exercise. Oxidative medicine is also useful as part of an intensive program to quickly establish blood sugar control in a poorly controlled diabetic.

WHERE TO FIND A DOCTOR

Although oxidative medicine has been commonly used in Europe for more than three decades, it is still relatively uncommon in the United States and many other parts of the world. I dare say that most physicians have probably never even heard of it.

Twice a year for the last ten years I have been teaching a course to train doctors in the use of these exciting treatments. To find a physician trained by me in oxidative medicine, go to the referral list at www.oxygen healingtherapies.com.

CHAPTER 14

Making It Happen for You

Always bear in mind that your own resolution
to succeed is more important than any one thing.
—ABRAHAM LINCOLN, 16TH PRESIDENT OF THE UNITED STATES (1809–1865)

A s I mentioned in Chapter 1, there are two different kinds of type 2 diabetes: the high-insulin type and the low-insulin type. The high-insulin type is the way diabetes almost always first presents itself. This is the stage of insulin resistance wherein the pancreas compensates for the ever-increasing resistance of the cells to the effects of insulin by manufacturing ever-increasing amounts of the hormone. It is in this phase that insulin levels begin to climb from an optimum of 5–10 microunits per milliliter (mU/ml) to over 15 mU/ml and even higher.

This form of diabetes can go on for months to years until eventually the islet cells (insulin-producing cells of the pancreas) start to become destroyed from being so overworked and the pancreas can no longer maintain producing the high levels of insulin needed by the body to overcome its insulin resistance. This is when the early phases of low-insulin diabetes show up, and it is manifested by declining (although often clinically classified as "normal") levels of insulin. As the number of islet cells continues to decline, it is usually not too long before a critical juncture is reached in which they become so depleted that the pancreas loses the ability to produce any insulin at all.

Of course, the sooner we catch your body in this whole process, the sooner we will be able to turn the process around, and the more effective many of our treatment strategies will be. This is particularly true of the low-insulin version of diabetes, because if it is not detected early enough, the usual outcome is that the patient will soon require insulin injections. Insulin injections are not the end of the world, but most people would agree that, all things being the same, it is better not to let the disease advance that far.

This chapter examines two patient cases, one an example of high-insulin diabetes (Tiffany's case), the other of low-insulin diabetes (Dale's case), and shows how each is treated slightly differently. In both cases there is a need to improve insulin sensitivity, but in the case of high-insulin diabetes, it is not necessary, indeed it is dangerous, to treat the patient with therapies designed to increase insulin output by the pancreas.

Tiffany and Dale's treatment programs offer examples of how the steps to success we have been discussing in Part II can be put into action. You will learn how Tiffany and Dale made it happen for themselves, but more importantly, in the process you will discover how easily you, too, can make it happen. Then, at the end of the chapter, you will find a description of "the perfect diabetic day," with a few tips on employing those keys to success in a regular routine.

HIGH-INSULIN DIABETES—TIFFANY'S CASE

Let's start with Tiffany. You might remember that it was Tiffany's first Bio-Energy Testing results that we used in Chapter 2 to demonstrate how the testing procedure could be used to treat and prevent the kind of energy deficit disorders that lead to diabetes. At the time she was tested, we had no idea that she actually had diabetes. I only ran her through the testing procedure to give her an idea of what it was like because she was going to be helping me put this book together.

In the process of demonstrating the testing to her, it became apparent that she, at the age of sixty-two, had diabetes. We were both quite surprised by this because, although she had developed a weight problem during the latter part of her life, up until the last twelve months Tiffany had been feeling great.

And even though she had noted a recent drop in her energy levels, she still felt herself to be way ahead of the norm. She told me at the time, "Having been a very high-energy person with great endurance all of my life, I can still outdo most people, but I know that the way I am feeling now is just not me." Furthermore, her annual visits with her physician failed to show anything abnormal on her routine testing.

Here's how her testing came out. Her two-hour glucose-tolerance test revealed that she had a severe case of diabetes with an almost total inability to metabolize glucose. Her hemoglobin A1c level of 9.2 percent confirmed the seriousness of the problem.

Her insulin level was 16 mU/ml, indicating that she had high-insulin diabetes. As you will recall, this is the first stage of diabetes, and is the one that is the easiest to cure. So far, this fact was about the only good news we had found. Finally, her cortisol levels were very low, indicating that her adrenal glands were in a state of exhaustion.

A synopsis of her Bio-Energy Testing, the complete results of which were reported in Chapter 2, revealed an abundance of information:

- Her Adrenal Factor was decreased at 95 (optimal > 100; that is, optimal is greater than 100), indicating a weakening adrenal gland function.

- Her M-Factor was decreased at 83 (optimal > 100), indicating decreased thyroid and/or adrenal function. Tiffany had been taking a very high dose of thyroid, which her blood test confirmed was excessive; therefore, her decreased M-Factor had to be due to an exhausted adrenal gland

- Her C-Factor was decreased at 76 (optimal > 100), indicating that even though she had been on a low-carbohydrate diet, it wasn't nearly low enough for her needs.

- Her Fat-Burning Factor was 74 (optimal > 100), indicating that not surprisingly she was not burning fat well. One of the main reasons for this is her decreased adrenal function.

- Her Fitness Factor was decreased at 72 (optimal > 100), indicating that at the age of sixty-two she had already lost a significant amount of her muscle mass. This fact alone will account for much of her insulin resistance.

- Her Heart Factor was 86 (optimal > 100), indicating that her heart was beginning to suffer from her lack of exercise.

- Her body composition indicated that she was about fifty pounds overweight, and figuring on the loss of one pound a week, it was probably going to be around a year before she could completely cure her problem.

- Her optimum caloric intake was 1,241 calories per day. This was a little more than 1,000 calories less than would have been predicted by a dietician using the standard reference tables, which only serves to indicate how seriously in error these tables can be.

- Her EQ, the measurement of her total aerobic energy output, was 91 (optimal>100), which was a real breath of fresh air. As bad as her diabetes was, with an EQ this good it was apparent that Tiffany was going to respond really well to therapy.

- Her optimal exercise zone was 140–150 beats per minute. This is important because exercise is going to play a critical role in getting her health back, and we need to be sure that she exercises correctly. For her, exercising at an intensity that keeps her heart rate between 140 and 150 beats per minute is just what the doctor needs to order.

Based on this information, I started Tiffany on a treatment program, as follows:

- To assist her liver, I placed her on QuickStart-DM.

- To improve her C-Factor, she was counseled to avoid all grains, sweets, fruits, legumes, and root vegetables.

- Her excessive thyroid medication was reduced to a more acceptable level.

- To improve her adrenal function and thus her M-Factor, she was placed on cortisol, licorice extract, DHEA, and pantothenic acid.

- To improve her Fat-Burning Factor, she was placed on lipoic acid, niacin, omega-3 oil capsules, L-carnitine, *Citrus aurantium*, L-tyrosine, and *Camellia sinensis* extract.

- To improve her insulin sensitivity, she was placed on high-dose chromium (3,000 mcg/day), *Galega officinalis*, and bitter melon.

- To improve her Fitness Factor, her Heart Factor, and her insulin sensitivity, she was placed on an exercise program consisting of walking for thirty minutes per day at a pace fast enough to keep her heart rate in her optimum exercise zone.

- To improve her weight control, she was placed on a diet constrained by her optimal caloric intake of 1,250 calories.

- To improve her aerobic energy production, she was placed on CoQ_{10}.

- She already had good habits regarding sleep and stress and so no therapy was needed there.

Tiffany was intentionally not started on medications such as the sulfonylureas or herbs such as *Gymnema sylvestre*. These treatments stimulate the pancreas to produce more insulin, which in her case would have worsened her prognosis. She was already making too much insulin. A lack of insulin was not what her problem was. Instead, what she needed was to improve her fat metabolism, increase her body's sensitivity to insulin, and increase her overall energy production.

Tiffany's Course

Within about two weeks of beginning her treatment program, Tiffany was already starting to feel more like her old self. She had more energy and she noticed that her exercise stamina had improved rather dramatically in even that short period of time. Furthermore, her blood sugar levels had started to get much closer to normal.

She was missing her carbs and wishing that she didn't need to be so compulsive about the exercise, but at the same time she knew that if she didn't stay on the program she would set herself up for a lot of misery down the line. In this light, carbohydrates didn't look nearly as attractive as they had before.

Four months later, Tiffany came in for her re-evaluation. Her fasting blood sugars, which had been 233 milligrams per deciliter (mg/dl), were now less than 120 mg/dl. This is considered to be normal. Her insulin level had dropped to 11 mU/ml, which is almost perfect. She had lost twenty-two pounds, indicating that her fat metabolism had kicked in. Her hemoglobin A1c was 6.7 percent. This was a dramatic improvement over the 9.2 percent of only four months before.

Best of all, her Bio-Energy Testing results indicated an improvement across the board. She was producing more energy and she was producing more of it from fat, the perfect recipe for recovery. Tiffany was well on the road to completely curing her condition. And best of all was the fact that she not only had become fully used to her new lifestyle, she was actually enjoying it.

She loved having more energy and less weight, and she especially was happy just knowing that she was turning her diabetes around. Four months were under her belt already, and all she needed to do to get where she wanted to be was to stay with the same program for another eight months. We decided not to change anything. There was no doubt in either one of our minds that diabetes was never going to be a problem for Tiffany as long as she made sure to keep her energy levels up, which she has done.

It's been almost two years now since she first turned off the road to diabetes and started heading in the direction of health and energy. And instead of becoming progressively less able to mange her weight and her blood sugars as would typically be the case, she actually weighs less and is having a much easier time keeping her blood sugar at nondiabetic levels.

LOW-INSULIN DIABETES—DALE'S CASE

I met Dale at a lecture I was giving. At that time Dale was fifty years old. He came up to me after the lecture and said, "Dr. Shallenberger, everything you said made complete sense to me. I have had diabetes for four years now, and I have asked my doctor many times about treatments other than medication for my condition. Other than to tell me to follow the ADA [American Diabetic Association] diet and exercise recommendations, he had nothing else to tell me. I know the ADA diet is a waste of time, because as soon as I got off of it on my own, I saw an immediate improvement in my energy levels as well as in my blood sugar levels."

Dale was the kind of patient that every physician wants to work with. He has a zest for life and a willingness to "do whatever it takes" to live better. He was very happily married and had already made his millions. There was nothing standing in his way except this diagnosis of diabetes. At Dale's first appointment here's what we found.

Unlike Tiffany, Dale had an extremely significant family history of diabetes. His father, his paternal grandfather, and both maternal grandparents all had diabetes. With this extensive history he should have been watched like a hawk by his physicians, who should have been compulsively doing everything they could to prevent Dale from ever getting diabetes. Instead, his doctors employed the "wait and see" attitude, which is so typical of the medical profession when it comes to preventable diseases.

Between the ages of forty and forty-five, Dale was allowed to gain over fifty pounds without his doctors ever saying anything. They didn't even look at his insulin levels in all this time. If it weren't for the fact that this kind of second-rate care is the current "standard of care," he would have the grounds for a malpractice case, in my opinion. But in our medical system, prevention is not considered all that important.

When Dale first learned of his diagnosis, he took things into his own hands. After learning how ineffective the ADA diet was, he went on a low-carbohydrate diet and started an exercise program. Within a matter of eight months he lost fifty pounds, and his blood sugars were starting to improve.

His doctor placed him on a sulfonylurea medication to boost his insulin levels without even checking his levels to see if this was needed. Since the levels were never checked, we can only hope that Dale started out with low-insulin diabetes, because if he started out with the high-insulin version, the medication his physician started him on may have worsened his condition by overworking his pancreas.

It is worth repeating here that the damage to the pancreas that results from overworking it is mediated by free-radical molecules, and to a large extent this damage can be prevented by taking enough antioxidant supplements, such as the vitamins C and E. Unfortunately and not surprisingly, however, Dale's physician never counseled him regarding antioxidant protection.

When the sulfonylurea medication was not effective by itself, his doctor then started adding in other medications. By the time I saw him, his medications had been increased to four, including one for hypertension, and his doctor had informed him that it was inevitable that within a certain amount of time he was going to need to go on insulin injections.

Here's what we found on Dale's first visit. First of all, consistent with the fact that a diabetic can never really trust how he feels to help him know how well he is doing, Dale felt great. He reported that his energy was good and that he had no complaints at all about his health. His evaluation, however, revealed an entirely different picture.

His hemoglobin A1c was 8 percent, revealing very poor control of his blood sugar. At this level it was almost certain that Dale would at some point develop many, if not all, of the complications of diabetes, such as blindness, kidney failure, heart disease, and neuropathy.

His fasting blood sugars were actually quite good, about 120–130 mg/dl on average, which is why one can't completely rely on them. Dale's main problem was not his fasting blood sugars, but the rise in blood sugar that comes after eating. Even after a low-carbohydrate meal he would often see an elevation in his blood sugar in excess of 300 mg/dl, due to the fact that his pancreas was just not able to produce very much insulin.

His insulin level was 6.1 mU/ml. Normally, I like to see a low insulin level like this in a patient, but seeing it in a patient with poorly controlled blood sugars who is already on a medication known to increase insulin output just indicates that the pancreas is getting very close to completely failing. If Dale's insulin levels were to get much lower than this, he would have had to go on insulin.

On the other hand, Dale's C-peptide levels were looking a little better. This was encouraging, because C-peptide is a marker in the blood that often gives a much better indication than insulin levels of whether or not pancreatic failure is imminent. With these C-peptide levels it was looking possible that we were treating him early enough to prevent pancreatic failure. At least that's what we were hoping. Here's what we learned from Dale's Bio-Energy Testing results:

- His Adrenal Factor was decreased at 94 (optimal>100), indicating a weakening adrenal gland function. Unfortunately, his physician never checked Dale's cortisol levels so we don't know what they were before.

- His M-Factor was significantly decreased at 78 (optimal>100), indicating decreased thyroid and/or adrenal function. Odds are fairly good that he had both.

- His C-Factor at 97 (optimal>100) was almost perfect, indicating that he had his carbohydrate intake down to an almost perfect level. Indeed, Dale virtually never ate carbohydrate anymore. With a C-Factor this good I did not need to counsel him on his diet. He already had that down.

- His Fat-Burning Factor was 74 (optimal>100), indicating that, not surprisingly, he was not burning fat well. One of the main reasons for this was his decreased thyroid and adrenal function.

- His Fitness Factor was decreased at 63 (optimal>100), indicating that at the age of fifty he had already lost a significant amount of his muscle mass. This fact alone will account for much of his insulin resistance.

- His Heart Factor was 80 (optimal>100), indicating that his heart was beginning to fail. The heart is a muscle, and even with exercise it will tend to weaken in the face of deficiencies of growth hormone and testosterone. As you will soon see, Dale turned out to be deficient in both of these hormones.

- His body composition was perfect. Dale had done an exceptional job on his own in getting his weight down to exactly where it needed to be.

- His EQ, the measurement of his total aerobic energy output, was extremely low at 77 (optimal>100). This low value gave him a biological age of sixty-two, which means that although he was only fifty, his body was producing energy no better than the average sixty-two year old. Dale was not too happy about this, but it did serve as a powerful motivational tool to inspire him to improve his energy dynamics.

- His optimal exercise zone was 110–130 beats per minute. This turned out to be very important because from it we learned that Dale had been wasting all his exercise time by exercising at levels that were inefficient and, in fact, harmful to him. At his trainer's advice, he had been spending most of his time exercising at a heart rate of 150. At this heart rate he was not only not burning any fat at all, but he was also dramatically increasing his rate of free-radical damage. In short, he was doing just about everything necessary to increase the likelihood of pancreatic damage and failure. Reining in his exercise would play a critical role in helping Dale protect his pancreas from any further damage and get his health back.

After seeing Dale's low Fitness Factor, I immediately ordered a hormone profile on him, which was very interesting. His levels of growth hormone were those typical of an eighty-five-year-old man, and he was also quite low on testosterone.

Based on Dale's Bio-Energy Testing and hormone profile results, I started him on a treatment program, as follows:

- To assist his liver, I placed him on QuickStart-DM.

- To improve his M-Factor, he was placed on a combination of the thyroid hormones T3 and T4 and the adrenal hormones cortisol and DHEA. In addition, to support his adrenal gland, he was placed on licorice extract, DHEA, and pantothenic acid.

- To improve his Fat-Burning Factor, he was placed on lipoic acid, niacin, omega-3 oil capsules, L-carnitine, *Citrus aurantium*, L-tyrosine, and *Camellia sinensis* extract.

- He was not placed on any medications for insulin sensitivity since he was already on two excellent drugs. Furthermore, I did take him off of his sulfonylurea medication and placed him on high-dose vitamin C and E, along with the amino acid N-acetylcysteine to help protect his pancreas from any further damage.

- In the hopes that his pancreas might be able to regenerate some of the islet cells that had been destroyed, I started him on *Gymnema sylvestre*.

- In order to improve further on his insulin sensitivity, we added vanadium and high-dose chromium, and also started him on regular intravenous oxidation therapy.

- To improve his Fitness Factor and his Heart Factor, he was placed on an exercise program consisting of walking fast enough to get his heart rate up to 110 and leaving it there for three minutes. Then he was to jog or run fast enough to get his heart rate up to 130 for one minute. He was to continue this form of interval training, alternating between these two heart rates for thirty to forty minutes, three to four days out of every week. The other three to four days, he was to employ resistance training using his heart rate according to the guidelines I discussed in the Chapter 8.

- He was also placed on a combination of growth hormone injections and testosterone injections in order to bring his hormone levels up to those typical of a forty-year-old man. Because growth hormone can sometimes worsen blood sugar control, Dale carefully monitored his sugars.

- To improve his very pathetic EQ, he was placed on a substantial dose (300 mg) of CoQ_{10}.

- Dale already had good habits regarding sleep and stress, so no therapy was needed there.

Dale's Course

For a person like Dale, adjusting to the above program was not much of an issue. He had already discovered in himself a strong determination combined with a commitment to self-discipline, so he was not intimidated by the idea of change. He just wanted to be healthy, and he didn't care what he had to do to accomplish that goal. Within a few weeks he was up and running on the entire program.

The next time I saw him was after four weeks, just to check on how things were going. He had adapted to everything and was continuing to feel great. Nothing surprising there.

He did report, however, that his fasting blood sugars had risen about ten to twenty points on average. I attributed this to the fact that I had taken him off his sulfonylurea medication and his body had not yet adapted to the change. I told him to continue to keep track of his fasting blood sugar levels and let me know if they continued to rise. I set the next visit for a full evaluation for four months later. Here are the results of that visit:

- His hemoglobin A1c had come down to 6.8 percent, which is considered to indicate good diabetic control. Although for many physicians this number might be acceptable, for me and Dale it was nowhere near where we needed it to be, which was in the nondiabetic zone of less than 6 percent. However, the fact that his hemoglobin A1c had responded so well was an excellent indication that his pancreas had not burned out, and that he might have made these changes in time to save him from the need for insulin injections.

- His fasting blood sugars were now back down to the levels of when he was on the sulfonylurea medication. This was another really good omen.

- His insulin levels and his C-peptide levels remained about the same. Again, this was a good sign.

- His testosterone levels were elevated. Because of this, we reduced the dose of the hormone about 30 percent. The new dose was likely to be just perfect, but we would continue to monitor levels until we were certain. I also checked his estrogen and his PSA levels just to be sure that the testosterone replacement was not creating any problems, and it wasn't.

- His growth hormone levels were just perfect, and so the dose of this hormone remained the same.

- Dale's Bio-Energy Testing results were much better. Every single one of his measurements had significantly improved. He was showing an increase in total energy production as well as increased fat metabolism. Happily enough for him, his biological age was now forty-five. From a biological standpoint he had become seventeen years younger in a matter of four months.

As a result of this excellent response to therapy, it was decided to just maintain the same program and have repeat evaluations every four to six months. Dale follows my advice to the letter, and now, as he is traveling down the highway of life, he is watching his diabetic condition in the rearview mirror.

In all likelihood Dale will always need to take medication, and to this extent he will never be cured of diabetes. However, since I have been following his case for over three years now, I can tell you that he has never needed to go on insulin and probably never will.

Furthermore, his blood sugars are controlled so well that his hemoglobin A1c is less than 6 percent. This is a nondiabetic level! He will never have any of the complications that diabetics are normally prone to, and will live a long, happy, and full life thanks to his love of life and his dedication to doing what it takes. Oh, and by the way, his blood pressure normalized after only six months, and he no longer requires any medication for this.

THE PERFECT DIABETIC DAY

Ever had a perfect day? Actually, many would argue that every day is perfect within its own context, and I would be the last person to disagree with that kind of philosophy. But when I am using this phrase, I mean "perfect" in the sense of following your goals and working those goals into the routine of your day so that you almost get to the point that you are doing them automatically.

Here is a list of some of the routine behaviors that many of my diabetic patients are using to make their lives easier and healthier.

Morning

- Drink 12 ounces of water.

- Check blood sugar and blood pressure.

- Take 1 scoop of QuickStart-DM along with $\frac{1}{2}$ teaspoon Super Fat, 1 tablespoon ground flaxseed, and 1 scoop of protein powder.

- Take medications, hormones, and supplements.

- On most days, don't eat breakfast. Occasionally breakfast with bacon and eggs, cheese, or plain yogurt. (Remember, those who take insulin will need to alter their doses accordingly.)

Noon

- Drink 12 ounces of water.

- For lunch have either a salad with meat and/or cheese or a meat and vegetable combination. Vegetable soup is also a possibility. Try having leftovers from the previous night. Eat slowly, and don't overeat.

2:00 P.M.

- Take 1 scoop of QuickStart-DM along with $\frac{1}{2}$ teaspoon Super Fat, 1 tablespoon ground flaxseed, and 1 scoop of protein powder.

- Take medications, hormones, and supplements.

- Drink two or more glasses of water during the rest of the afternoon.

Evening

- Drink 12 ounces of water.

- For supper have a meat entrée (possibilities include fish, seafood, poultry, beef, and so on—all hopefully grain-free), a large salad, and a substantial amount of vegetables. Finish supper no later than three hours before you plan to sleep. Eat slowly, and don't overeat.

Bedtime

- Make sure that you go to bed early enough to get at least eight hours of sleep. If you are behind in your sleep for whatever reason, get enough extra sleep to make up for your debt.

- Take your bedtime medications, hormones, and supplements.

Exercise

Exercise for at least thirty minutes per day. I believe that exercise in the late afternoon is the best time for two reasons: it will enhance sleep, and this is the time when blood sugars start to creep up due to decreased adrenal activity. Avoid exercising before sleep as it will probably keep you awake.

Stress

Dealing with stresses is vital to success. If you think stress is playing too much of a role in your life, then practice breath meditation for about fifteen minutes before you start your day, and again toward the end of your day.

At first look, getting into a daily routine that enhances your health may be a little daunting in this twenty-four-hour-convenience world of ours, but it has never been more important. And the great thing about establishing a daily routine is that it is like magic, because once things get to be routine, they get to be habitual, and all of a sudden they become so easy that it seems that they are doing you instead of you doing them. Don't forget the words of one of our greatest presidents, which I quoted at the beginning of this chapter: if you want to make it all happen for yourself, remember that "your own resolution to succeed is more important than any one thing."

Appendix A

Resources

PHYSICIANS

To find a physician in your area who is likely to be familiar with many of the concepts in this book, try these websites:

www.acam.org—the website of The American College for Advancement in Medicine, a nonprofit medical society dedicated to preventive/nutritional medicine.

www.holisticmedicine.org—a site offering referrals to holistic medicine practitioners and suppliers in the United States.

www.bioenergytesting.com—the official website for Bio-Energy Testing. Besides including a list of clinics offering Bio-Energy Testing, this site also posts new information regarding energy production.

www.oxygenhealingtherapies.com—a site that posts a referral list of doctors trained by Dr. Shallenberger in oxidative medicine.

BIO-ENERGY TESTING

To obtain the name of a facility in your area offering Bio-Energy Testing, visit the website www.bioenergytesting.com, or call toll-free 1-866-376-0610.

DR. SHALLENBERGER'S SUPER IMMUNE QUICKSTART-DM AND SUPER FAT

As discussed in Chapter 9, QuickStart-DM is a comprehensive nutritional supplement I specially designed to help my patients with diabetes take better care of their livers. Super Fat is another supplement that I recommend taking with QuickStart-DM as part of an energy-boosting breakfast and midday smoothie.

QuickStart-DM

Take one scoop in the morning and another in the early afternoon. Two scoops contain the following:

30,000 IU beta-carotene

100 mg niacin (B_3)

10,000 IU vitamin A

300 mg pantothenic acid (B_5)

2,000 mg vitamin C

100 mg vitamin B_6 (pyridoxine)

400 IU vitamin E (d-alpha)

1,000 mcg methylcobalamine (B_{12})

1,000 mg Hesperidin Bioflavonoid Complex

1,000 mcg folic acid

500 mcg biotin

600 mg magnesium (citrate)

10 mg manganese (amino acid chelate)

6 grams Spirolina pacifica

300 mg potassium (citrate)

750 mg L-glutamine

200 mcg selenium (selenate)

250 mg N-acetylcysteine

1,200 mcg chromium (picolinate)

50 mg zinc (picolinate)

5 grams psyllium husks

2 mg copper (amino acid chelate)

5 grams stabilized rice bran

100 mg vitamin B_1 (thiamine)

5 grams soy protein isolate

50 mg vitamin B_2 (riboflavin)

5 grams whey protein (undenatured)

5 grams cinnamon powder

160 mg *Galega officinalis* extract (standardized to 20% guanylhydrazine)

200 mg R-lipoic acid

740 mg Mormodica charantia (4:1 extract)

Super Fat

Take $^1/_2$ teaspoon with QuickStart-DM in the morning and another in the early afternoon. One teaspoon contains the following:

3 cubic centimeters (cc) fish oil concentrate

1cc wheat germ oil

1cc flax oil

135 mg mixed tocopherols (containing 20% gamma-tocopherol)

15 mg lycopene

50 mg CoQ_{10}

750 IU vitamin D_3

To purchase QuickStart-DM and/or Super Fat, please visit the website www.bioenergytesting.com. Alternatively, these products can be purchased by calling toll free 1-866-376-0610.

APPENDIX B

Is Your Patient Exercising Too Hard to Be Healthy?

Abstract of a 2004 Article
Published in *Townsend Letter for Doctors*

Aerobic exercise is a documented and well-accepted measure to decrease incidence of degenerative disease, increase quality of life, and extend life span. However, exercising above anaerobic threshold is known to increase free-radical production and exhaust both antioxidant buffering and acid-base buffering capabilities. Both of these phenomena are known to increase the rate of aging as well as tissue and organ degeneration. This study examines whether or not the two most popular current methods of predicting anaerobic threshold—the formula that is anaerobic threshold heart rate = $0.8 \times (220 - \text{age})$, or the determination of the heart rate at which the subject feels breathlessness and muscle pain—are safe methods to use in prescribing an exercise regimen.

The true anaerobic threshold heart rate of nineteen patients of various ages was measured using Bio-Energy Testing, and then compared to the anaerobic threshold heart rates predicted by either the above formula or when the subject reported breathlessness and muscle pain. Both methodologies were found to be unreliable in 100 percent of patients tested.

Exercise programs prescribed on the basis of this formula and these symptoms would result in 90 percent of patients exercising above their aerobic capacity. Such exercise causes dangerously high levels of oxidant stress and increases the burden of acid levels in the tissues, known as mesenchymal acidosis.

For the full article, please see Frank Shallenberger, M.D., "Is Your Patient Exercising Too Hard to Be Healthy?" *Townsend Letter for Doctors* August/September 2004, pp. 97–99.

Notes

Introduction

1. Suzanne Rostler, "Experts Fear Type 2 Diabetes Epidemic in U.S. Children," *Reuters Health*, September 8, 2000.

2. See the website www.mercola.com/2003/jun/25/child diabetes.htm.

Chapter 2

1. T.M. Wilson and H. Tanaka, "Meta-Analysis of the Age-Associated Decline in Maximal Aerobic Capacity in Men: Relation to Training Status," *Am J Physiol Heart Circ Physiol* 2000;278:829 34.

Chapter 6

1. R. Endevelt, D.R. Shahar, "Omega-3: The Vanishing Nutrient Beyond Cardiovascular Prevention and Treatment," *Journal of the Israeli Medical Association* April 2004;6(4):227–32.

2. C. Popp-Snijders, J.A. Schouten, R.J. Heine, J. van der Meer, A. van der Veen, "Dietary Supplementation of Omega-3 Polyunsaturated Fatty Acids Improves Insulin Sensitivity in Non-Insulin-Dependent Diabetes," *Diabetes Res* Mar 1987;4(3):141–47.

3. G.A. Colditz, "Epidemiology of Breast Cancer. Findings from the Nurses' Health Study," *Cancer* Feb 15, 1993;71(4 suppl):1480–9.

4. G.A. Boissonneault, C.E. Elson, M.W. Pariza, "Net Energy Effects of Dietary Fat on Chemically Induced Mammary Carcinogenesis in F344 rats," *J Natl Cancer Inst* Feb 1986;76(2):335–8.

Chapter 7

1. K.M. Fairfield, R.H. Fletcher, "Vitamins for Chronic Disease Prevention in Adults: Scientific Review," *JAMA* June 19, 2002;287(23):3116–26. Review, erratum in: *JAMA* Oct 9, 2002;288(14):1720.

2. A.D. Mooradian et al., "Micronutrient Status in Diabetes Mellitus," *American Journal of Clinical Nutrition* 1987;45(5):877–95.

3. M. La Selva, E. Beltramo, F. Pagnozzi, E. Bena, P.A. Molinatti, G.M. Molinatti, M. Porta, "Thiamine Corrects Delayed Replication and Decreases Production of Lactate and Advanced Glycation End-Products in Bovine Retinal and Human Umbilical Vein

Endothelial Cells Cultured Under High Glucose Conditions," *Diabetologia* Nov 1996;39(11):1263–68.

4. B. Barbiroli, C. Frassineti, P. Martinelli, S. Iotti, R. Lodi, P. Cortelli, P. Montagna, "Coenzyme Q_{10} Improves Mitochondrial Respiration in Patients with Mitochondrial Cytopathies. An In Vivo Study on Brain and Skeletal Muscle by Phosphorous Magnetic Resonance Spectroscopy," *Cell Mol Biol (Noisy-le-grand)* Jul 1997;43(5):741–49.

5. T. Kishi, H. Kishi, T. Watanabe, K. Folkers, "Bioenergetics in Clinical Medicine. XI. Studies on Coenzyme Q and Diabetes Mellitus," *J Medicine* 1976;7(3/4):307–21.

6. Y. Shigeta et al., "Effect of Coenzyme Q_{10} Treatment on Blood Sugar and Ketone Bodies of Diabetics," *J Vitaminology* 1966;12:293–98.

7. G. Paradies, F.M. Ruggiero, M.N. Gadaleta, E. Quagliariello, "The Effect of Aging and Acetyl-L-Carnitine on the Activity of the Phosphate Carrier and on the Phospholipid Composition in Rat Heart Mitochondria," *Biochim Biophys Acta* Jan 31, 1992;1103(2):324–6.

8. B. Barbiroli, R. Medori, H.J. Tritschler, T. Klopstock, P. Seibel, H. Reichmann, S. Iotti, R. Lodi, P. Zaniol, "Lipoic (Thioctic) Acid Increases Brain Energy Availability and Skeletal Muscle Performance as Shown by In Vivo 31P-MRS in a Patient with Mitochondrial Cytopathy," *J Neurol* Jul 1995;242(7):472–7.

9. S. Jacob, P. Ruus, R. Hermann, H.J. Tritschler, E. Maerker, W. Renn, H.J. Augustin, G.J. Dietze, K. Rett, "Oral Administration of RAC-Alpha-Lipoic Acid Modulates Insulin Sensitivity in Patients with Type 2 Diabetes Mellitus: A Placebo-Controlled Pilot Trial," *Free Radic Biol Med* Aug 1999;27(3–4):309–14.

10. R.A. Anderson, N. Cheng, N.A. Bryden, M.M. Polansky, J. Chi, J. Feng, "Elevated Intakes of Supplemental Chromium Improve Glucose and Insulin Variables in Individuals with Type 2 Diabetes," *Diabetes* Nov 1997;46(11):1786–91.

11. G. Boden, X. Chen, J. Ruiz, G.D. van Rossum, S. Turco, "Effects of Vanadyl Sulfate on Carbohydrate and Lipid Metabolism in Patients with Non-Insulin-Dependent Diabetes Mellitus," *Metabolism* Sep 1996;45(9):1130–5.

12. K. Baskaran, B. Kizar Ahamath, K. Radha Shanmugasundaram, E.R. Shanmugasundaram, "Antidiabetic Effect of a Leaf Extract from *Gymnema sylvestre* in Non-Insulin-Dependent Diabetes Mellitus Patients," *J Ethnopharmacol* Oct 1990;30(3): 295–300.

Chapter 8

1. R.S. Paffenbarger Jr, R.T. Hyde, A.L. Wing, C.C. Hsieh, "Physical Activity, All-Cause Mortality, and Longevity of College Alumni," *N Engl J Med* Mar 6, 1986;314(10):605–13.

2. S.N. Blair, H.W. Kohl III, R.S. Paffenbarger Jr, D.G. Clark, K.H. Cooper, L.W. Gibbons, "Physical Fitness and All-Cause Mortality. A Prospective Study of Healthy Men and Women," *JAMA* Nov 3, 1989;262(17):2395–401.

3. M. Pahor, J.M. Guralnik, M.E. Salive, E.A. Chrischilles, S.L. Brown, R.B.Wallace, "Physical Activity and Risk of Severe Gastrointestinal Hemorrhage in Older Persons," *JAMA* Aug 24–31, 1994;272(8):595–9.

4. J.A. Laukkanen, T.A. Lakka, R. Rauramaa, R. Kuhanen, J.M. Venalainen, R. Salonen, J.T. Salonen, "Cardiovascular Fitness as a Predictor of Mortality in Men," *Arch Intern Med* Mar 26, 2001;161(6):825–31.

5. M. Babyak, J.A. Blumenthal, S. Herman, P. Khatri, M. Doraiswamy, K. Moore, W.E. Craighead, T.T. Baldewicz, K.R. Krishnan, "Exercise Treatment for Major Depression: Maintenance of Therapeutic Benefit at 10 Months," *Psychosom Med* Sep–Oct 2000;62(5):633–8.

6. J.G. Lim, H.J. Kang, K.J. Stewart, "Type 2 Diabetes in Singapore: The Role of Exercise Training for Its Prevention and Management," *Singapore Med J* Feb 2004;45(2): 62–8.

7. I. Janssen, A. Fortier, R. Hudson, R. Ross, "Effects of an Energy-Restrictive Diet with or without Exercise on Abdominal Fat, Intramuscular Fat, and Metabolic Risk Factors in Obese Women," *Diabetes Care* Mar 2002;25(3):431–8.

8. F.B. Hu, T.Y. Li, G.A. Colditz, W.C. Willett, J.E. Manson, "Television Watching and Other Sedentary Behaviors in Relation to Risk of Obesity and Type 2 Diabetes Mellitus in Women," *JAMA* Apr 9, 2003;289(14):1785–91.

9. V.R. Soman, V.A. Koivisto, D. Deibert, P. Felig, R.A. DeFronzo, "Increased Insulin Sensitivity and Insulin Binding to Monocytes After Physical Training," *N Engl J Med* Nov 29, 1979;301(22):1200–4.

Chapter 9

1. K. Grungreiff, D. Reinhold, "Liver Cirrhosis and "Liver" Diabetes Mellitus Are Linked by Zinc Deficiency," *Med Hypotheses* 2005;64(2):316–7.

2. S.K. Taneka et al., "Assessment of Copper and Zinc Status in Hair and Urine of Young Women Descendants of NIDDM Parents," *Biol Trace Elem Res* 1998;62(3): 255–64.

3. K.M. Fairfield, R.H. Fletcher, "Vitamins for Chronic Disease Prevention in Adults: Scientific Review," *JAMA* June 19, 2002;287(23):3116–26. Review, erratum in: *JAMA* Oct 9, 2002;288(14):1720.

Chapter 10

1. William Dement, *The Promise of Sleep* (New York: Dell Publishing, 1999), back cover and 262–63.

2. Verlyn Klinkenborg, "Awakening to Sleep," *The New York Times Magazine* January, 5, 1997.

3. Quoted in Stanley Coren, *Sleep Thieves* (New York: Simon & Schuster, 1996), 36.

4. C.F. Reynolds III, D.J. Kupfer, C.C. Hoch, P.R. Houck, J.A. Stack, S.R. Berman, P.I. Campbell, B. Zimmer, "Sleep Deprivation as a Probe in the Elderly," *Arch Gen Psychiatry* Nov 1987;44(11):982–90.

5. G.A. Christos, "Is Alzheimer's Disease Related to a Deficit or Malfunction of Rapid Eye Movement (REM) Sleep?" *Med Hypotheses* Nov 1993;41(5):435–9.

6. K. Spiegel, R. Leproult, E. Van Cauter, "Impact of Sleep Debt on Metabolic and Endocrine Function," *Lancet* Oct 23, 1999;354(9188):1435–9.

7. T. VanHelder, J.D. Symons, M.W. Radomski, "Effects of Sleep Deprivation and Exercise on Glucose Tolerance," *Aviat Space Environ Med* Jun 1993;64(6):487–92.

8. N.T. Ayas, D.P. White, W.K. Al-Delaimy, J.E. Manson, M.J. Stampfer, F.E. Speizer, S. Patel, F.B. Hu, "A Prospective Study of Self-Reported Sleep Duration and Incident Diabetes in Women," *Diabetes Care* Feb 2003;26(2):380–4.

9. K. Spiegel, E. Tasali, P. Penev, E. Van Cauter, "Brief Communication: Sleep Curtailment in Healthy Young Men Is Associated with Decreased Leptin Levels, Elevated Ghrelin Levels, and Increased Hunger and Appetite," *Ann Intern Med* Dec 7, 2004; 141(11):846–50.

Chapter 12

1. L.J. Valenta and A.N. Elias, "How to Detect Hypothyroidism When Screening Tests Are Normal. Use of the TRH Stimulation Test," *Postgrad Med* Aug 1983;74(2):267–74.

2. S. Yamashita, H. Namba, S. Nagataki, "Thyroid and Radiation," *Nippon Naibunpi Gakkai Zasshi* Nov 20, 1993;69(10):1035–43.

3. Ronald Klatz and Robert Goldman, *Stopping The Clock* (New Canaan, CT: Keats Publishing, Inc., 1996), 58.

4. D.L. Coleman, R.W. Schwizer, E.H. Leiter, "Effect of Genetic Background on the Therapeutic Effects of Dehydroepiandrosterone (DHEA) in Diabetes-Obesity Mutants and in Aged Normal Mice," *Diabetes* Jan 1984;33(1):26–32.

5. Ibid.

6. D. Kalman, *Curr Therapeut Res* 2000;61:435–42.

7. G. De Pergola, "The Adipose Tissue Metabolism: Role of Testosterone and Dehydroepiandrosterone," *International Journal of Obesity* 2000;24(supplement 2):S59.

8. P. Diamond et al., "Metabolic Effects of 12-Month Percutaneous Dehydroepiandrosterone Replacement Therapy in Post-Menopausal Women," *Journal of Endocrinology* 1996;150(supplement):S43–S50.

9. D.T. Villareal, J.O. Holloszy, "Effect of DHEA on Abdominal Rat and Insulin Action in Elderly Women and Men: A Randomized Controlled Trial," *JAMA* Nov 10, 2004; 292(18):2243–8.

10. H. Kawano, H. Yasue, A. Kitagawa, et al., "Dehydroepiandrosterone Supplementation Improves Endothelial Function and Insulin Sensitivity in Men," *Journal Clinical Endocrinology and Metabolism* July 2003;88(7):3190–95.

11. K. Dhatariya, M. Bigelow, S. Nair, "Effect of Dehydroepiandrosterone Replacement on Insulin Sensitivity and Lipids in Hypoadrenal Women," *Diabetes* 2005;54:765–69.

12. M.A. Boyanov, Z. Boneva, V.G. Christov, "Testosterone Supplementation in Men with Type 2 Diabetes, Visceral Obesity and Partial Androgen Deficiency," *Aging Male* Mar 2003;6(1):1–7.

13. R.K. Stellato, H.A. Feldman, O. Hamdy, E.S. Horton, J.B. McKinlay, "Testosterone, Sex Hormone Binding Globulin, and the Development of Type 2 Diabetes in Middle-Aged Men: Prospective Results from the Massachusetts Male Aging Study," *Diabetes Care* Apr 2000;23(4):490–94.

14. M.O. Thorner, M.L.Vance, E. Horvath, K. Kovacs, "The Anterior Pituitary" in *Williams Textbook of Endocrinology*, 8th ed. (Philadelphia: W.B. Saunders Company, 1992), 230.

15. Y.J.H. Janssen, M. Frolich, F. Roelfrsema, "A Low Starting Dose of Genotropin in Growth Hormone Deficient Adults," *J Clin Endocrinol Metab* 82:129–35.

Index

About the Author

Frank Shallenberger, M.D., has devoted his thirty-year professional career to understanding the fundamentals of what keeps us well. To this end, he has used an approach in his medical practice that integrates the best of alternative, natural-healing medicine with the best of conventional medicine.

He is a pioneer in the clinical application of oxidative medicine, a modern discipline that emphasizes the profound importance of oxygen and energy production in health and longevity. Using a revolutionary technology that he invented and patented known as Bio-Energy Testing, he is able to measure the energy production of patients, and improve it to more youthful levels.

Dr. Shallenberger is the founder and medical director of the Nevada Center of Alternative and Anti-Aging Medicine in Carson City, Nevada, a facility that attracts patients from all over the country. He is board certified in Anti-Aging Medicine, and has served as a Clinical Instructor in Family Medicine at the University of California School of Medicine in Davis. In 2001 he was a keynote speaker at the First International Learning Conference on Anti-Aging Medicine in Monte Carlo, a global gathering of health professionals interested in applying anti-aging strategies.

Dr. Shallenberger is the lucky father of four fantastic children, and is grandfather to three. His extended family includes a joyous dachshund, a stubborn horse, two haughty llamas, and ten productive chickens. He is an avid backpacker, sailor, and cyclist. He has won numerous cycling events and garnered silver medals in the Nevada State Mountain Bike Championship Series and the Northern California Time Trials.

He aims to keep himself and his patients young and energetic for a long, long, long, long time.